P9-CDA-140

Sharon — 972
Elizabeth — 972-548-1099
Kristen — 972-548-1117
Sheryl —
Chris — 214-354-3511 (cell)
972-359-7387

FIRST PLACE BIBLE STUDY

Giving

CHRIST FIRST PLACE

Gospel Light

FIRST PLACE™

Gospel Light is an evangelical Christian publisher dedicated to serving the local church. We believe God's vision for Gospel Light is to provide church leaders with biblical, user-friendly materials that will help them evangelize, disciple and minister to children, youth and families.

It is our prayer that this Gospel Light resource will help you discover biblical truth for your own life and help you minister to others. May God richly bless you.

For a free catalog of resources from Gospel Light, please contact your Christian supplier or contact us at 1-800-4-GOSPEL or www.gospellight.com.

PUBLISHING STAFF
William T. Greig, Publisher
Dr. Elmer L. Towns, Senior Consulting Publisher
Pam Weston, Senior Editor
Patti Pennington Virtue, Associate Editor
Jeff Kempton, Editorial Assistant
Hilary Young, Editorial Assistant
Kyle Duncan, Associate Publisher
Bayard Taylor, M.Div., Senior Editor, Biblical and Theological Issues
Dr. Gary S. Greig, Senior Advisor, Biblical and Theological Issues
Barbara LeVan Fisher, Cover Designer
Samantha A. Hsu, Designer

ISBN 0-8307-2864-3
© 2001 First Place
All rights reserved.
Printed in the U.S.A.

All Scripture quotations, unless otherwise indicated, are taken from the *Holy Bible, New International Version*®. Copyright © 1973, 1978, 1984 by International Bible Society. Used by permission of Zondervan Publishing House. All rights reserved.

Other version used is:

Phillips— The New Testament in Modern English, Revised Edition, J. B. Phillips, Translator. © J. B. Phillips 1958, 1960, 1972. Used by permission of Macmillan Publishing Co., Inc., 866 Third Avenue, New York, NY 10022

Any omission of credits is unintentional. The publisher requests documentation for future printings.

CAUTION
The information contained in this book is intended to be solely informational and educational. It is assumed that the First Place participant will consult a medical or health professional before beginning this or any other weight-loss or physical fitness program.

CONTENTS

FOREWORD

My introduction to Bible study came when I joined First Place in March of 1981. I had been in church since I was a small child, but the extent of my study of the Bible had been reading my Sunday School quarterly on Saturday night. On Sunday morning, I would listen to my Sunday School teacher as she taught God's Word to me. During the worship service, I would listen to our pastor as he taught God's Word to me. Digging out the truths of the Bible for myself had frankly never entered my mind.

Perhaps you are right where I was back in 1981. If so, you are in for a blessing you never dreamed possible. As you start studying the truths of the Bible for yourself, you will see God begin to open your understanding of His Word. Bible study is one of the nine commitments of the First Place program. The First Place Bible studies are designed to be done on a daily basis. Each day's study will take approximately 15 to 20 minutes to complete, but you will be discovering the deep truths of God's Word as you work through each week's study.

There are many in-depth Bible studies on the market. The First Place Bible studies are not designed for the purpose of in-depth study. They are designed to be used in conjunction with the other eight commitments of the program to bring balance into our lives. Our desire is for each member to begin having a personal quiet time with God each day. This time alone with God would include a time of prayer, Bible reading and Bible study. Having a quiet time is a daily discipline that will bring the rich rewards of balance, something we all need.

A part of each week's study is the Bible memory verse for the week. You will find a CD at the back of this Bible study that contains all 10 of the memory verses for the study. The CD has an upbeat tempo suitable for use when exercising. The songs help you to easily memorize the verses and retain them for future reference. If you will memorize Scripture as you study, God will use His Word to transform your life.

Almost every First Place member I have talked with about the program says, "The weight loss is wonderful, but the most important thing I have received from my association with First Place is learning to study God's Word."

God bless you as you begin this exciting journey toward a balanced life. God will richly bless your efforts to give Him first place in your life. Remember Matthew 6:33: "But seek first his kingdom and his righteousness, and all these things will be given to you as well."

Carole Lewis
First Place National Director

INTRODUCTION

The First Place Bible studies were developed to be used in conjunction with the First Place weight-loss program. However, the studies could also be used by anyone who desires to learn more about God's Word and His will, with the added bonus of learning more about living a healthy lifestyle.

A Balanced Life

First Place is a Christ-centered health program, emphasizing balance in the physical, mental, emotional and spiritual areas of life. The First Place program is meant to be a daily process. As we learn to keep Christ first in our lives, we will find that He is the One who satisfies our hunger and our every need.

God's Word contains guidelines for maintaining our physical well being, equipping us mentally to make right choices, providing emotional stability to handle everyday circumstances as well as crisis situations, and growing spiritually as we deepen our relationship with Him.

The Nine Commitments

The First Place program has nine commitments that will help you draw closer to the Lord and aid you in establishing a solid, consistent and healthy Christian life. Each commitment is a necessary and important part of the goal of First Place to help you become healthier and stronger in all areas of your life—living the abundant life He has planned for each of us. To help you achieve growth in all four areas, First Place asks you to keep these nine commitments:

1. Attendance
2. Encouragement
3. Prayer
4. Bible Reading
5. Scripture Memory Verse
6. Bible Study
7. Live-It Plan
8. Commitment Record
9. Exercise

The Components

There are six distinct components to this Bible study to aid you in bringing balance to your life. These components include the 10-week Bible study, 6 Wellness Worksheets, 2 weeks of menu plans, the leader's discussion guide, 13 Commitment Records and the Scripture memory CD.

The Bible Study

Each week of each 10-week Bible study is divided into five daily assignments with days six and seven set aside for reflections on the week's lesson. The following guidelines will help make your study more enjoyable and profitable:

- Set aside 15 to 20 minutes each day to complete the daily assignment. It's best not to attempt to complete a week's worth of Bible study in one day.
- Pray before each day's study and ask God to give you understanding and a teachable heart.
- Keep in mind that the ultimate goal of Bible study is not for knowledge only but also for application and a changed life.
- First Place suggests using the *New International Version* of the Bible to complete the studies.
- Don't feel anxious if you can't seem to find the *correct* answer. Many times the Word will speak differently to different people, depending upon where they are in their walk with God and the season of life they are experiencing.
- Be prepared to discuss with your fellow First Place members what you learned that week through your study.

Wellness Worksheets

The informative and interactive Wellness Worksheets have been developed by Dr. Jody Wilkinson at the Cooper Institute in Dallas, Texas. These worksheets are intended to help you understand and achieve balance in all four areas of your life: physical, mental, emotional and spiritual. Your leader will assign specific worksheets as At-Home Assignments throughout the 13-week session.

Menu Plans

The two-week menu plans were developed especially for First Place by Chef Scott Wilson. Each menu is meant to simplify meal planning and include food exchanges. These meals are based on the MasterCook software that uses a database of over 6,000 food items, which was prepared using United States Department of Agriculture (USDA) publications and information from food manufacturers.

Leader's Discussion Guide

This discussion guide is provided to help the First Place leader guide a group through this Bible study. It provides information for the leader to prepare for each weekly group meeting.

Commitment Records

Thirteen Commitment Records (CRs) are provided in the back of this Bible study. For your convenience these have been printed on perforated paper so that you may easily remove them from the book and carry them with you through each week as you keep your First Place commitments. Directions for filling out the CRs precedes those pages.

Scripture Memory CD

Since Scripture memory is such a vital part of the First Place program, the Scripture memory CD for this study is included in the back inside cover. The verses for this study are set to music that can be listened to as you work, play or travel. The CD can be an effective tool as you exercise since the first verse is set to music with a warm-up tempo, the next eight verses are set to workout tempo, and the music of the last verse can be used for a cooldown.

GIVING CHRIST FIRST PLACE

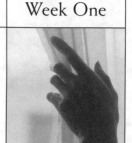

MEMORY VERSE

*But seek first his kingdom and his righteousness,
and all these things will be given to you as well.*
Matthew 6:33

When embarking upon a journey toward better health, we need to seek God's help and claim His promises. In Matthew 22:37 we discover the place God wants to hold in our lives—*first place*. What a challenge! Loving God halfheartedly is not enough. He wants complete commitment, and through that commitment to Him your life will be forever changed.

In this week's study, you'll have the opportunity to search your heart and examine your life. Are there areas of your life you have failed to surrender to Christ? If Christ is not first place in your thoughts, plans and actions, what is?

DAY 1: *Time for What You Seek First*

Matthew 6:33 puts the pattern for Christian living in a nutshell: Seek first the kingdom of God. In your busy life you cannot do everything. However, the thing you *can* decide is what to do first. What you choose first, over time, takes first place in your life.

If you look at the entries in your calendar or checkbook for the past month, you might be surprised by what has been first place in your life lately.

➤ List areas to which you find yourself giving the most time and effort.

*Kids
work
housework
Wishing I was doing something else @ the time
I'm doing something.*

God knows that things other than spiritual priorities tend to become the focus of our lives. Your checkbook and calendar will remind you of this fact.

➤ In Matthew 6:25 Jesus mentioned some of the things that divert our attention from His priorities in our lives. What are those things?

your life, food, drink, body, clothing

Jesus wasn't saying that what you eat, drink or wear is not important; He simply stressed that you need not worry about them. These concerns must never take first place in your life. Instead, Jesus has challenged you to learn some simple lessons about God's provision.

➤ According to Matthew 6:26-30, what does God want you to learn from the birds and flowers?

They do not worry about their food or shelter. God takes care of them & they are splendid.

When you see the lessons of His provision for the birds and flowers, you will begin to understand how God knows and meets your needs. Philippians 4:19 also reminds you of His promise. He didn't say He would meet some or a few of your needs, but all your needs.

And My G will supply all your needs according to His riches in glory in Christ Jesus

➤ Do you believe this promise applies to you? ☑ Yes ☐ No

➤ What needs do you have in your life now that you can turn over to God? *what to eat, how to proceed w/ this weight loss, job, whole life*

As Christians, the desire to give Christ first place in every area of our lives must be foremost. *Saying* Christ is first and *living* with Christ in first place are different matters. When Christ comes first, your life will change. You will make decisions based on new commitments. You will schedule time based on new priorities.

Use this week's memory verse to keep this commitment in focus.

Listen to the CD while exercising. Display the verse in the bathroom and/or kitchen and read it each time you are in that room. Memorizing Scripture will reinforce your commitment to keep Christ in first place and direct your thoughts and actions toward Christ and His kingdom.

Thank You Lord, for the promise to meet my needs through Your Son, Jesus.

Lord, help me to trust You and give You first place in my life this week.

DAY 2: *God's Promise . . . Your Choice*

Consider Matthew 6:25-27. When Jesus spoke about "these things" in Matthew 6:33, He was referring to what He said in the verses that preceded verse 33, beginning at verse 25. He offered a choice: 1) worry about these things *or* 2) seek His kingdom. God has promised that we will receive what we need. In spite of this, most Christians continue to worry rather than simply claim this promise. Worry is an affront to God. He told us He would supply all our needs, and He knows what we need even before we ask.

In Matthew 6:28-30, Jesus continued to teach about not worrying about the things of life. Worry is different from being concerned. God wants you to be concerned about others, situations, what is happening in your life and your relationships with others. Pray earnestly about those things, but don't worry and fret over them. If the situation is one over which you have no control, give it to God—He does have control.

⟫ What are the things that cause you worry?

John, weight, lonely $, Kerry, Tracy, Sean, bills.

⟫ How much time and energy do you give each week to worrying about the things God has promised to provide for those who seek His kingdom first? *Too much*

➤ What could you do when you find yourself worrying about something? *Seek God – Pray – Turn it over to God*

When Jesus taught his disciples how to pray in Matthew 6:9-13, part of the prayer focused on the kingdom of God: "Your kingdom come, your will be done on earth as it is in heaven." You will glimpse God's kingdom when His will is done on Earth as it is in heaven.

➤ How would your life change if you could invest your emotional energy in spiritual priorities, rather than wasting it on worrying? How could you have more time for prayer, Bible study, exercise, witnessing or serving Him? *Set specific time for these things – no excuses – do not give myself permission to slack.*

In Matthew 21:22 we find another wonderful promise from God. When you pray about the things that cause you to worry and when you believe in God's faithfulness, He will provide what you need. What changes would come in your life this day if you asked God to use you to accomplish His will this day in your part of the world—at school, the office, the store or your own home? Allow His kingdom to break through on Earth today through you.

Remember the Serenity Prayer:

> *God, grant me the serenity to accept the things I cannot change*
> *Courage to change the things I can*
> *And the wisdom to know the difference.*
> —Reinhold Neibuhr, 1926

As you pray today, list in your prayer journal the details of your worries or concerns and turn them over to Him. Repeat the memory verse in your prayer, telling God that you are willing to seek His kingdom first. Ask Him to help you trust Him more.

Lord, help me to trust You and to seek You and Your kingdom first.

Lord, help me to focus my energy on things that will make a difference for Your kingdom.

DAY 3: *The Priorities of the Kingdom of God*

Romans 14:17 tells us three things that *are* and two things that *are not* priorities in the kingdom of God.

⤳ List the three things that are priorities in the kingdom of God.

1. *Righteousness*
2. *peace*
3. *joy in the Holy Spirit*

⤳ List the two things that are not priorities.

1. *eating*
2. *drinking*

Did you notice that two of these items focus on our physical lives and three of them focus on our spiritual lives? The Bible does not teach that your physical life is unimportant or that it is unnecessary to provide for yourself and those who depend on you.

⤳ What do 2 Thessalonians 3:10 and 1 Timothy 5:8 tell us about taking care of responsibilities and physical needs?

If anyone is not willing to work then he is not to eat, either. But if anyone does not provide for his own & esp. for thes) he has denied the faith - is worse than an unbeliever.

While you need to focus on spiritual priorities, you also need to care for your own physical needs and the needs of others. The challenge comes as you attempt to live responsibly without allowing daily pressures to consume all your time and energy. It is our experience that when you nurture your spiritual life, you will find the added emotional energy you need to live in this demanding physical world.

First Corinthians 10:31 gives us a guideline for transforming the activities of everyday life into a lifestyle focused on God and spiritual priorities. Whatever you do during the day, whether eating, drinking or playing, do it all for God's glory.

➤ Write a statement that expresses what "for the glory of God" means to you. *Know tto is pleasing to A. In his will —*

➤ If you wanted to live today for the glory of God, what would you do? *Seek to be more Christlike —*
Praise, Pray, Serve.
Lam. Mind of heart & words/mouth morith pleasing to God

➤ How would this change the way you normally live your life? *Spend more time Praising, less time being negative*

➤ To what degree are you experiencing God's righteousness, joy and peace? *On & off*

➤ To what extent are you glorifying Him through your eating and exercise habits? *doing much better than before —*

Do you lack the energy needed to be all you can be through the First Place commitments? Use the following prayers to ask for God's help.

Lord, help me to balance my time and energy to meet the demands of my life today.

Lord, help me to glorify You in all that I do and say this day.

DAY 4: *Commitments to Giving God First Place*

Luke 9:23 contains three commitments we must make if we want to follow Christ with the kingdom of God as our top priority.

➤ What are the commitments Jesus asked His disciples to make?

1. *deny himself (yourself)*
2. *take up cross daily*
3. *follow Jesus*

➤ Describe one area in which you need to deny yourself so you can follow Christ more fully.

— food, benging, choices made —

➤ Considering your cross as a positive personal ministry you do for other people, what could you do today to take up your cross?

➤ What is one step you need to take in following Christ that you might have been reluctant to do until now?

Trust Jesus to help me w/ my eating + exercise.

➤ In Luke 9:57-62, the cost of following after Jesus is described. What were some of the excuses given by those who said they wanted to follow Him?

Take care of family, say good bye to those @ home

➤ What excuses do people use when asked to do something for their church such as teach a class, volunteer in the nursery, visit the sick, answer the telephone, work in the library or any of the many other tasks related to carrying out God's business?

Scheduling problems, family parents

When Jesus told us to take up our cross and follow Him, He meant we were to follow Him wherever He would go. He healed the sick, ministered to those in need, taught His disciples, prayed for sinners, and He depended on His Father to supply all His needs.

If you want to follow Jesus and be like Him, you must be willing to commit yourself to doing the tasks of furthering His kingdom. Seek Him first, and He will help you do all things through Him. Remember Philippians 4:13. Your source of strength is Christ.

Review this week's memory verse.

Lord, help me, today, to put my past behind me, take up my cross and follow You.

Lord, show me how to please You in everything I do, including in what I eat and drink.

DAY 5: *Your Spiritual Connection and Evidence*

Matthew 5:16 describes a time when Jesus told His disciples to let their lights shine so that others could see their works and praise their Father in heaven.

≫ Fill in the blanks in the following paragraph:

Jesus assumed that His disciples would live lives that attracted attention. Others would see the _god works_ they did and pay attention to their lives. But Jesus wanted His disciples to do more than attract attention. He wanted people to see their good deeds and _glorify your Father in heaven_.

In most cases, people will not make the connection between your good deeds and your Father in heaven unless you help them. You will have to tell them that the reason you live as you do is because of the difference Christ has made in your life. Only then will they glorify God because of your deeds.

≫ How would you respond if a coworker or friend said, "You are such a disciplined person! I don't know how you have so much self-control!"?

≫ The following verses describe some of the priorities and commitments that indicate you have given Christ first place. Look up each verse and match the verse with the key phrase.

Scripture		Characteristic in Our Lives
a. 1 Samuel 15:22	_A_ 1.	A desire and willingness to obey God
b. Proverbs 3:9,10	_C_ 2.	Offering yourself to God as a living sacrifice
c. Romans 12:1	_B_ 3.	Giving to God from material possessions
d. Romans 13:8	_D_ 4.	Loving others on an ongoing basis
e. 1 Thessalonians 5:17	_E_ 5.	An ongoing lifestyle of prayer

Based on these verses, how would you evaluate the degree to which Christ is first place in your life right now? Check the box beside each characteristic that best expresses the degree to which it has developed in your life:

Characteristic in My Life	Strong	Average	Weak
I desire to know and obey God.	☑	☐	☐
I offer myself to God as a living sacrifice.	☐	☐	☑
I give to God from my material possessions.	☑	☐	☐
I love others on an ongoing basis.	☑	☐	☐
I sustain a lifestyle of prayer.	☐	☑	☐

In your prayer journal write a prayer for another person in your First Place group and ask God to help this person with whatever needs or struggles he or she is facing. Then write a prayer for a non-Christian who is in your life—such as a neighbor, coworker or family member—and ask the Lord to let the light of God's love in your life shine to others.

 Lord, give me the opportunity to help a friend, family member or coworker make a spiritual connection through my life.

God, give me the wisdom to explain the connection between the way I live and the fact that Jesus is first place in my life.

DAY 6: *Reflections*

You've been studying the Bible for five days; this may be a new experience for you or it may already be a daily part of your life. In either case these studies will help you establish new patterns for your life. Bible study requires a greater priority on the spiritual level of your life than the physical elements of other commitments.

The Reflection section at the end of each week will introduce a powerful spiritual resource—praying through the Scriptures. Whether this is your first or fifth Bible study for First Place, this section will help you overcome those things in your life that have become strongholds. If you are not familiar with praying through Scripture, this section will teach you how. For repeaters, this section will be a refresher and will reiterate those things you've learned.

Praying through Scripture is the process of taking a verse and praying it back to God in your own words. Beth Moore's book *Praying God's Word*[1] explains the process.

You can learn much about letting God be in control and overcoming your own strongholds through Beth Moore's own testimony.

> *I've been educated in the power of God and His Word through field trips of my own failure, weakness, and past bondage . . . I didn't discover what a vital part of my liberation this approach has been until long after I had begun practicing it. I suddenly realized it was no accident that I was finally set free from some areas of bondage that had long hindered the abundant, effective, Spirit-filled life in me.*[2]

Beth tells us that a stronghold may be an addiction, an unforgiving spirit toward a person who has hurt you, or despair over loss; and it demands so much of your emotional and mental energy that your abundant life is strangled. You, too, can break down the spiritual strongholds in your life as you pray through the Scriptures.[3]

The process isn't complicated: You take a particular verse and pray that verse to the Lord, personalizing the words. The following are examples of praying Scripture. Ask the Lord to reveal the strongholds in your life as you pray each one.

Lord, help me overcome the strongholds in my life. I long for You to be first. I want to seek first Your kingdom and Your righteousness. Thank You for your promise to give me the other things I need (see Matthew 6:33).

Father, when Your words come to me, help me to eat them; make them my joy and my heart's delight, for I bear Your name, O Lord God Almighty (see Jeremiah 15:16).

God, through the victories You give, may Christ's glory be great (see Psalm 21:5).

DAY 7: *Reflections*

The key to overcoming strongholds can be found in 2 Corinthians 10:3-5. Consider carefully the meaning of the words. You can pray this Scripture by saying,

> *Lord, You've said I live in the world, but I do not wage war as the world does. My weapons are not the weapons of the world. On the contrary, they have divine power to demolish strongholds. I can demolish arguments and every pretension that sets itself up against the knowledge of God; and I take captive every thought to make it obedient to Christ. Thank You in advance for working in my life. Amen.*

Before you can tackle the spiritual strongholds in your life, you need to identify the battlefield. As a believer in Jesus, the enemy is waging a constant, personal battle against you and the primary battlefield is your mind.

Your mind is the control center of your being. Satan tries to make you believe that he is powerful and that you are powerless, and he will try to put destructive and discouraging thoughts in your mind. But you are not powerless; you have God's Holy Spirit living in you. Repeat these words: Nothing is bigger or more powerful than God! The strongest addiction or your worst habit can be overcome through the power of the living God.

The primary goal of your spiritual warfare is found in the verses you just prayed: You need to demolish every argument and pretension that sets itself up against the knowledge of God. You must take your thoughts captive and be obedient to Christ.

As you complete this first week of Bible study, repeat the memory verse. Keep your Scripture memory cards close at hand to help you review. Try saying the verse aloud to a family member or use it in conversation. Each time you use the verse, God will plant this verse more firmly in your mind and heart.

The journey to seek God first begins with a single step. The completion of this first week is a step of progress on that journey. Rejoice at the opportunity to give Christ first place.

Father God, please help me to keep in mind that my struggle is not against flesh and blood, but against the rulers, against the powers of this dark world and against the spiritual forces of evil in the heavenly realms (see Ephesians 6:12).

Lord, I know I have nothing to fear from my strongholds because You have given me a spirit of power and of love and of a sound mind (see 2 Timothy 1:7).

Lord, thank You for Your protection. Help me to be sober and vigilant because the devil walks around like a lion, seeking whom he may devour. Help me be steadfast in the faith (see 1 Peter 5:8).

Heavenly Father, help me to seek first Your kingdom and Your righteousness, for then all these other things will be given to me (see Matthew 6:33).

Notes
1. Beth Moore, *Praying God's Word* (Nashville, TN: Broadman and Holman, 2000).
2. Ibid., p. 2.
3. Ibid., p. 3.

GROUP PRAYER REQUESTS   TODAY'S DATE: 3/21/03

NAME	REQUEST	RESULTS

*Member's Guide - What's Big Deal about H₂O
p129-131
Study Gods word a heart
P 23-25
Understanding out Gain
+ obenty Part I —
pg 111-114*

LORD, TEACH US TO PRAY

MEMORY VERSE

*If you believe, you will receive whatever
you ask for in prayer.*

Matthew 21:22

Lining up Plan pg 31-73

Prayer is one of the daily commitments of the First Place program. A vital part of your spiritual life is your communication with God through prayer. Through the First Place Bible study, you will learn to pray using Scripture as the basis of your prayers.

On one occasion, Jesus' disciples asked Him, "Lord, teach us to pray" (Luke 11:1). Jesus didn't scold or rebuke them for not knowing how to pray. He responded gently, guiding them into new insights about talking with God.

Jesus wants to teach you how to pray. The Bible is the text. In this week's study, you'll learn about people who prayed effectively. You'll discover patterns for praying, what the Bible teaches about how to pray, why you pray and what to expect when you pray.

DAY 1: *What You Believe About God*

⇒ What does Hebrews 11:6 say to you? *& w/o faith it is impossible to please God, because anyone who comes to him must believe that he exists and that he rewards those who earnestly seek him.*

Prayer acknowledges that God exists. When you pray, you seek God; you admit that you need God's help. The key question is: Do you believe God hears your prayer and will help you? *If do in his will — how do you know if your requests are in his will.*

➣ After reading the following verses, write the main idea of each verse in your own words. Look for ideas common to all four.

Matthew 21:21,22 *Have faith, do not doubt — All things are possible - if you believe you will receive whatever you ask for in prayer.*

Mark 9:23 *Everything is possible for him who believes*

Mark 11:22-24 *Believe, forgive others so your sins will be forgiven. Then you will receive what you ask for in prayer.*

James 1:6 *Ask believe do not doubt, because he who doubts is like a wave of the sea, blown + tossed by the wind*

When you pray, believe and don't doubt. Each of these verses affirms this principle. You can pray with confidence because you have a powerful and loving God. When you place your faith in God, you stand on a strong foundation. Faith demands a focus. Your focus as a Christian is Jesus Christ. As you learn to know Jesus more fully, it becomes easier to place faith in Him. You discover that He is faithful. You can trust Him. Your faith will grow stronger.

Many Scriptures dealing with prayer contain two parts: a condition and a promise. You cannot claim the promise if you do not meet the condition.

Read each of the following verses and complete the chart.

	CONDITION	PROMISE
Matthew 21:21,22	*If you believe, have faith, do not doubt*	*you will receive whatever you ask for in prayer*
Mark 11:24	*must believe that you will receive it*	*It will be yours.*
Mark 11:25	*forgive others if you holding anything against anyone (forgive)*	*God in heaven may forgive you your sins*
John 15:7	*Remain in Christ Gospel and my words remain in you*	*ask whatever you wish & it will be given to you*
1 John 3:21,22	*hearts not condemn us have confidence before J. & we have confidence Obey his commands & do what pleases him*	*receive what we ask*

Pray with confidence. God knows your needs and will work all things together for your good today.

Thank you, Lord, for the promise to hear and answer my prayers when I pray and believe.

Father, You told me that You will not break Your covenant with me. Give me the faith and strength I need to keep the covenant I made with You on the day of my salvation.

DAY 2: *Prayer—A Priority in Your Life*

"Very early in the morning, while it was still dark, Jesus got up, left the house and went off to a solitary place, where he prayed" (Mark 1:35). This passage gives you a clear picture of Jesus' prayer life. From His example you can learn the three principles of prayer. The first principle explains why prayer is one of the commitments of the First Place program; the other two follow naturally.

A Commitment to Pray

➤ Mark 1:21-34 describes Jesus' activities the day before He rose early
to pray. How do you think Jesus felt at the end of the previous day?

Drained, very tired.

➤ Are you surprised He got up early to pray after a day like that?
Would you have done the same thing? Why or why not?

*I am guilty of not praying as I should.
Alot of times I try to sleep instead of
being + doing the things I know I should
do.*

A Time to Pray

➤ In this situation Jesus prayed early in the morning. On other occasions, He prayed in the evening, and sometimes He prayed all night.
When is the best time for you to pray?

Evening / middle of day

A Place to Pray

➤ Jesus found a place where He could be alone. People demanded Jesus'
time and attention constantly. He struggled to find places where He
could be alone. What place can you set aside where you can be alone
with God?

My Bedroom

One of your commitments in First Place is spending time in prayer. If
prayer was so important in the life of Jesus, it should also be a priority in
our lives. Throughout the New Testament you will find Jesus praying. His
prayer in the Garden of Gethsemane just before His betrayal shows you
how to pray for God's will, even in the darkest of circumstances.

➤ In Mark 14:35-41 Jesus again goes off to pray alone. How many times did Jesus pray?

2 or 3

➤ For what did He pray (see v. 36)?

God's will to be done.
Take this cup from me

➤ What was the condition Jesus put in His prayer?

Not what I will but what A's will

Jesus knew the power of God, and He knew the pain and humiliation that was to come. If there had been any other way for your salvation, God would have spared His Son. They both knew the answer. Jesus prayed that His Father's will would be done. He stood ready to go to the cross.

Spend time with God every day. Commit yourself to that prayer time, and you will find that you, too, will say with confidence, "Nevertheless, not my will, but Yours be done."

Make a commitment now to find a place for prayer and to set aside a few minutes every day to spend with God.

➤ Check the following commitments you are willing to make.

☑ Commitment: I commit myself to pray each day.

☑ Time: The time of day I will pray is _*before bedtime / or middle of day*_

☑ Place: The place I have chosen where I can be alone each day in prayer is _*my Bedroom - /Kitchen table / front family room*_

Heavenly Father, I commit myself to pray just as You prayed, seeking God's will in my life, rather than my own.

Precious Lord and Savior, remove the obstacles that keep me from spending time with You each day.

DAY 3: Four Dimensions of Prayer

Many people think prayer only involves asking God for things. The Bible teaches there are at least four dimensions to prayer. Use the A-C-T-S acrostic to remember them.

Adoration: Express your love to God for who He is.

Confession: Seek God's forgiveness for sin in your life.

Thanksgiving: Express your thanks to God for what He has done.

Supplication: Seek God's answers for your needs and the needs of others.

➤ Read the following verses in your Bible and match each verse with the dimension of prayer it describes:

a. Psalm 9:1, 2   _A_   1. adoration

b. Psalm 100:4   _C_   2. confession

c. 1 John 1:9   _B_   3. thanksgiving

d. 1 John 5:14,15   _D_   4. supplication

➤ Evaluate your own prayer life based on each of these four dimensions. Circle a number on each line below to indicate how strong or how weak you think each dimension of prayer is in your life now:

Adoration	very weak	1	2	3	4	(5)	very strong
Confession	very weak	1	(2)	3	4	5	very strong
Thanksgiving	very weak	1	2	3	4	(5)	very strong
Supplication	very weak	(1)	2	3	4	5	very strong

➤ Practice using these four dimensions by writing a brief prayer for each.

A for *adoration*: I express my love to God for who He is.

I love you Lord

C for *confession*: I ask God's forgiveness for sin in my life.

Please forgive my faults and repeated sins I lift up to you now.

T for *thanksgiving*: I express my love to God for what He has done.

[handwritten:] all thing are possible thru you L. Thank you for your unfailing love and patience.

S for *supplication*: I seek God's answers for my needs:

[handwritten:] Lord thank you that you have all things in my life already mapped out. Help me to look to you & not myself — God's word is a light to my path & a lamp to my feet

Father, help me to express my love to You through prayer. Guide me in expressing my thoughts, ideas and concerns to You.

DAY 4: *More Than Words*

Many Christians feel awkward while learning to pray. We want to say the right words because we fear that God won't listen unless we use the right words. If you have ever had doubts about your prayers, the Bible offers good news!

After reading Romans 8:26,27 check the following boxes that express the good news:

☑ God understands our weakness, even our weakness in prayer.

☑ God's Holy Spirit, living in us, helps us pray for the right things.

☑ God listens to our thoughts, deepest longings and the desires of our hearts.

☑ We can sit silently before the Lord, trusting that He knows our desires.

The amazing truth is that He does all these things and so much more. God wants to talk with you more than you could ever want to pray. Through the Holy Spirit's work in your life, God enables you to have an ongoing conversation with Him. Some times words come easily in prayer. At other times, especially in times of crisis and pain, you do not know what to pray.

⟫ How can Matthew 6:8 reassure you when words fail?

God knows what we are or want even before we ask.

Even when words won't come, God knows your heart. Simply sit in silence in God's presence and allow your heart to speak for you. Relax and focus on God's presence. Thank Him for being with you and knowing your needs. Let the Holy Spirit make your silence a prayer to the Lord.

You have learned that prayer has a condition as well as a promise. One condition you must meet is to do what God says you must do. Then you can claim His promise and trust Him to do what He promised.

⟫ What is the promise found in Philippians 4:6,7?

The peace of G which transcend all understanding, will guard your hearts and your minds in Christ Jesus.

With so many promises from God concerning your prayers, you can pray with confidence that God hears your petition, or you can sit silently knowing that God hears your heart. What a joy and comfort this is to a believer.

Review this week's memory verse. Repeat it to yourself. The verse is short and easy to remember. Think of it each time you pray.

Lord, help me to pray with confidence, realizing that You know my every thought and desire before I utter a word and that You will answer when I pray believing Your Word.

Lord, I know that I can seek Your will with any request and that You will answer out of the abundance of Your great riches.

DAY 5: *Prayer Protection*

Some passages on prayer make it sound as if God is Santa Claus, waiting to give us anything we want—no matter what the consequences may be. Fortunately, truths in other verses protect us from Santa Claus prayers!

➤ What does 1 John 5:14,15 tell us about the prayers God hears and answers? *Ask anything according to his will he hears us.*

The principles in this verse provide the context in which we must understand prayer. God gives clear-cut conditions to go along with His promises. He will hear and answer our prayers when we pray according to His will.

After the completion of the Temple in Jerusalem the Lord appeared to Solomon and warned him what would happen if the people were disobedient. He then gave Solomon a condition and a promise for answered prayer in 2 Chronicles 7:14.

➤ What is the condition and promise found in 2 Chronicles 7:14? *If my people who are called by my name, will humble themselves + pray + seek my face and turn from their wicked ways, then will I hear from heaven and will forgive their sin and will heal their land.*

➤ How does this apply to you today?
① Humble yourself by admitting your sin
② Pray to L asking for forgiveness
③ Seek God continually
④ Turn from sinful behavior

God wants to give you the desires of your heart, but He also demands that you be obedient to Him and worship Him. The conditions He sets forth for your prayers keep you from praying for the wrong things or for the wrong reasons.

➤ Do you consider God's will a limitation on prayer that you wish He had not included? Why or why not?
No - always want to be in God's will - on the right path - He knows all -

➤ Would you want God to answer every prayer that you or anyone else in the world prayed, without any limitation? What problems might result if He did? *Chaos*

God answers prayers according to His will. God's will includes His wisdom—He knows all things. God's will includes His power—He can bring good out of any situation. God's will includes His love—He walks with us through everything.

Whether you pray for others in your group, for family and friends or for yourself, pray for the Lord to work out the solutions according to His will. That's the way Jesus taught His disciples to pray and that's the way He prayed.

➤ What was the prayer example set by Jesus in Matthew 26:39?

If this is the way Jesus Himself prayed, then how can you do anything less?

Lord, help me to seek Your will in my life and to pray according to that will.

God, I know You are the creator of the universe and that You can do all things. Help me to trust You to work out any situation that may arise in my life.

DAY 6: *Reflections*

You are continually learning that Bible study requires a greater priority on the spiritual level of your life than the physical elements of other commitments. The same is true with your prayer life.

Last week you were introduced to a powerful spiritual resource—praying through the Scriptures. This week you have learned how to pray according to God's will. The studies gave you an acrostic that is easy to remember when you pray. *A* for adoration, *C* for confession, *T* for thanksgiving and *S* for supplication offer a way to use the dimensions of prayer. Write this *ACTS* acronym in the front of your prayer journal and refer to it when you pray until it becomes a habit.

The following verses are samples of using Scripture to pray in these four dimensions:

> **A***doration*: Psalm 98:4
> **C***onfession*: James 5:16
> **T***hanksgiving*: Psalm 106:1
> **S***upplication*: Ephesians 6:18

James 5:16 and Ephesians 6:18 remind us to pray for one another. Knowing that others are praying for you will give you peace and comfort in times of trouble.

Whatever the hold is on your life, God can help you overcome it. Allow Him to free you from bondage whether it be related to your health, relationships with others, despair, resentment or an unforgiving spirit. God wants you to be balanced emotionally, physically, mentally and spiritually. Using His Word to pray through memorized Scripture will set you free.

 Help me, Lord, to take Your yoke upon me and learn from You, for You are gentle and humble in heart, and I will find rest for my soul (see Matthew 11:29).

Father, I call to You, and You will answer me and tell me great and unsearchable things I do not know (see Jeremiah 33:3).

God, I come to You in prayer and ask You now to let Your peace, that transcends all understanding, guard my heart and my mind in Christ Jesus (see Philippians 4:7).

DAY 7: REFLECTIONS

This week's memory verse states that if you believe, you will receive whatever you ask for in prayer. Remember that this doesn't mean that you can pray for just anything and it will happen. God's will must be included as a part of the conditions. God's will may not be exactly what you would like or plan, but His plan is in your best interests. In the garden Jesus prayed: "May this cup be taken from me. Yet not as I will, but as you will" (Matthew 26:39). God's will was done, and Jesus was crucified—for our sakes!

Are you ready for God's will to be done in your life? If you are, then "delight yourself in the LORD and he will give you the desires of your heart. Commit your way to the LORD; trust in him and he will do this: He will make your righteousness shine like the dawn" (Psalm 37:4-6). This is another condition of prayer. Remember the verses you studied this week that set forth the conditions and then the promises of prayer. The conditions concern having faith and seeking God's will.

Using Scripture in prayer both puts to use the weapons of warfare and meets the conditions of prayer. Delighting yourself in the Lord and committing your way to Him by using His Word when you pray will give you the answers you seek. God answers all prayers. Humble yourself, pray, seek His face and turn from your sin. Then He will hear from heaven and heal you (see 2 Chronicles 7:14).

As you complete your second week of Bible study, repeat the memory verse. Keep your Scripture cards close at hand to help you review. Each time you use the verse, God plants it more firmly in your mind and your heart.

Father God, turn my heart toward your statutes and not toward selfish gain. Turn my eyes away from the worthless things of this world and preserve my life according to Your Word (see Psalm 119:36,37).

Answer me when I call to You, O my righteous God. Give me relief from my distress and be merciful to me. Hear my prayer, O Lord Most High (see Psalm 4:1).

Lord God, I know that without faith it is impossible to please You. I believe in You and I know that You will reward those who earnestly seek You. Help me to seek You with all my heart and soul (see Hebrews 11:6).

Heavenly Father, I claim Your promise that if I pray
believing, I will receive whatever I ask for in prayer. Help me
to always seek Your will when I pray (see Matthew 21:22).

GROUP PRAYER REQUESTS   TODAY'S DATE: 3/28/03

NAME	REQUEST	RESULTS
Chris	Camille, Lesley, Gary,	
Kristen		
Sheryl		

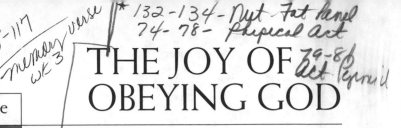

(handwritten margin notes) Eating
Pg Habits Inventory Part II
Inventory Part II
124–128
Pg 115–117
memory verse wk 3
* 132–134 – Nut Fat Panel
74–78 – Physical act
79–86
act Pyramid

THE JOY OF OBEYING GOD

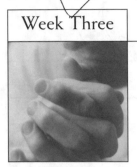

MEMORY VERSE

Whoever has my commands and obeys them,
he is the one who loves me. He who loves me
will be loved by my Father, and I too will love him
and show myself to him.

John 14:21

God expects us to obey Him. Not only our actions but even our thoughts and desires must be aligned with God's commands. God is serious about our obedience.

In this week's study you'll have an opportunity to examine what the Bible says about living a life of joyful obedience. You'll discover some incredible truths about what God will do in the life of one who obeys Him. You'll also learn about the consequences of living a disobedient life. Plus, you'll have the opportunity to evaluate your life to see how fully you are obeying God. Based on that evaluation, you'll be able to see what steps you'll need to take to follow Jesus in joyful obedience.

DAY 1: *Learning Obedience from Jesus*

If you want to learn anything well, find a master teacher—one who has mastered the skill or subject you want to learn. The same principle holds if you want to learn how to obey God. Fortunately, we have *the* Master Teacher to follow: Jesus. While He lived on Earth, Jesus always obeyed His heavenly Father. He modeled the way we should live in obedience.

➤ Luke 22:39-46 describes a night in Jesus' life when He struggled to obey God. How did Jesus express His personal desires to God?

He prayed earnestly *(handwritten answer)*

➤ What did Jesus want more than the fulfillment of His own personal desires? *God's will be done*

➤ Do you think that His attitude of submission to His Father's will made it easy for Jesus to face what was about to take place? Explain your answer. *no easy but able to go on.*

➤ This passage shows us Jesus agonizing in prayer, struggling to obey God. What did God do to encourage and help Jesus face what was coming? *Sent an angel from heaven to strengthen him.*

Ultimately, Jesus obeyed His Father unto death. Obeying God isn't easy and it wasn't easy for Jesus. During Christ's agonizing struggle, the Father sent angels to encourage and strengthen Him.

In 1 John 3:21,22 two principles—answered prayer and obedience—are linked. Obedience, then, becomes a condition for answered prayer.

➤ What is your confidence before God in prayer based on? *That David has and answer my prayers.*

Sometimes when God answers prayer, the answer isn't what you want to hear or have happen; but in your obedience to His will, God remains faithful and will help you accept His will over your own desires. Answered prayer remains a great mystery. You don't earn God's answers. You can't force God to answer prayer. Perhaps God entrusts answered prayers to people who have demonstrated that they want what God wants. God knows that those who obey Him and strive to please Him will use the answers to prayer to further serve and please Him.

From Jesus' prayer in the garden, we can learn four important concepts for prayer and obedience.

- Express your desires to God in prayer.
- Set aside what you want if it conflicts with what God wants.
- Don't expect life to be easy if you are obeying God.
- Expect God to strengthen you as you obey Him.

Dear Lord, give me an obedient spirit and help me to set aside my own desires when I pray.

Father, I pray for Your strength as I strive to follow Your will for my life.

DAY 2: *The Truth Obedience Reveals*

A well-known minister asked his congregation to consider if a trial were held to settle the issue as to whether or not they were Christians, would there be enough evidence to say they were, or would the case be dismissed for lack of evidence? What type of evidence establishes or demonstrates that you are a Christian?

➣ 1st John 2:3-6 presents four if-then statements. Write the missing half of each statement as needed to complete the idea.

IF	THEN
we obey his commands	We know we have come to know him.
We do not do what God commands	*is a liar & the truth is not in him*
We obey God's word	*Gods love is made complete in him*
we walk as Jesus did	We know that we are in Him.

These verses should be an encouragement for you. They show you exactly what must be done and then give the results. If you cannot say you are seeking to obey God, then you must question your true commitment to Him. Do you know for sure that you are a Christian and will go to heaven when you die? Check the box that best describes your answer:

☑ I know for sure I am a Christian.

☐ I don't know if I am a Christian, but I want to be certain if that is possible.

☐ I'm not a Christian, but I would like to become one.

If you have checked the second statement, talk to your First Place leader, a Christian friend or another group member. He or she will be able to provide guidance.

If you checked the third statement, you can acknowledge Jesus as the rightful Lord of your life and confess your sins to Him right now. When you have done this, contact your pastor or a Christian friend and tell him or her about your decision so that he or she can encourage you and help you grow in your faith.

➤ In looking at prayer from God's perspective, what would be the difference between His response to the prayer of a person who lives a life of obedience and the prayer of a person who lives to please only self?

➤ After reading the following passages, explain what each says about obedience.

Job 36:11

They will spend the rest of their days in prosperity and their years in contentment

Matthew 7:21

Only he who does the will of God

1 John 2:17

world & its desires pass away but the men who does the will of the God lives forever.

1 John 3:22

recieve what ever we ask because we obey his commands & do what pleases him

Heavenly Father, I commit myself to You and pray that You will help me to be obedient unto Your will.

Precious Lord and Savior, come in and be a part of every area of my life.

DAY 3: *Joyful Obedience*

What is the motivation behind your obedience to God? Is your obedience based on negative thoughts or reactions, or is your obedience based on the love God shows for you? Below are three negative and three positive ideas concerning obedience to God. Which ones have you experienced?

Negative

☐ I'll obey God because He will punish me if I don't.

☐ If I obey God, He will make me do things that will make me miserable.

☐ I guess I'll obey God. I owe Him that much.

Positive

☐ I'll obey God because He gives me so much in return.

☐ If I obey God, I'll experience His richest blessing.

☐ I'll obey God because of what Jesus did for me on the cross.

Reluctant obedience describes how many Christians respond to the challenge of obeying God. The Bible, however, presents a positive picture of the obedience that should characterize your life. If you checked any of the positive ideas above, you are experiencing the joy that comes from obedience.

→ After reading the following verses, match each positive obedience principle with the verse from which the principle is drawn.

God's Truth	Positive Obedience Principles
a. Deuteronomy 26:16	_C_ 1. I've evaluated my life and decided to obey God.
b. Psalm 40:8	_A_ 2. I'm careful to obey God.
c. Psalm 119:59,60	_A_ 3. With all my heart and soul, I long to obey God.
	_B_ 4. I desire to obey God.
	____ 5. I'm ready and willing to obey God immediately
	_C_ 6. I'm not reluctant to obey God.

→ What is the common thread that binds Isaiah 55:12, John 16:22 and Galatians 5:22 together? *fruit of Spirit - joy, peace*

Joy. peace, song
Joy, rejoice

In view of the joy found in salvation and obedience to God, learn to obey Him joyfully and not reluctantly.

Dear Lord, restore the joy of salvation as I learn obedience and seek to do Your will.

Father God, give me the desire to love You and serve You with all my heart.

DAY 4: *Your Rock-Solid Foundation*

How do you respond when you encounter challenges in your life? Do you hold up well or do you crumble? The key might be your spiritual foundation. By obeying God, you can build a solid foundation for your life.

➤ In Luke 6:46-49, Jesus told a story to illustrate this principle. What is the comparison He made in this parable?

house built on rock vs sand (no foundation)

Think about your own experience in obeying God and write your insights after each statement.

➤ When you obey God, how do you feel about yourself?

Great

➤ When you obey God, how do you feel about life in general?

Good

➤ When you obey God, how do you feel about your ability to handle challenging situations?

Confident.

God communicates His plans for you and teaches you the principles on which you should build your life.

➤ According to Jeremiah 29:11-13, what are God's plans for your life and what does God promise when you call upon Him and seek Him with all your heart? *prosper, hope, future*

You can claim God's promise through your obedience to Him. You have a choice: to obey or disobey. When you obey, you express your love for God. As you obey God, your choice anchors your life on His solid foundation.

Lord, help me to build my life on the solid foundation of Your love.

Lord, Your Word promises that You will listen when I pray. Hear my prayer and instill in me the desire to be obedient to You.

DAY 5: *Discovering Your Obedience Limit*

Have your ever said no to the Lord—or at least tried to? Since Jesus is Lord of all and the rightful Lord of your life, your response to Him must be "Yes, Lord."

Jesus demonstrated this attitude while He was on Earth in His relationship with His heavenly Father. Jesus is our teacher, and you must learn from Him so you can live as He did. God wants you to constantly be ready to say "Yes, Lord" as He leads you.

➤ Hebrews 5:8 is an example of Jesus' obedience to His heavenly Father. To what extent did Jesus obey His Father? *perfectly even under great trial*

➤ What does the phrase "he learned obedience" mean to you?

process is a [handwritten]

➤ Philippians 2:5-8 is another example of Jesus' total obedience to His heavenly Father. What was Jesus' ultimate act of obedience?

Death on a Cross [handwritten]

➤ In what areas of your life are you obeying God? List some specific areas of your life where you know God's will and are now working to bring your life in line with His plans.

— Submissive to husband [handwritten]
— working on Bible Study [handwritten]
—

➤ Are there any areas in your life where you are being disobedient? Are these areas with which you have had struggles in the past? Identify any area in your life where you know what God wants you to do, but you just don't want to obey at this time.

Eating choices, exercise, forgiveness, [handwritten]

Think about times you have responded to God's leadership in your life by saying "Yes, Lord." Then think about the times when the issues or concerns in a situation may have prompted you to say "No, Lord." If you ask Him, God will give you the strength and desire to do His will. God stands ready to answer a prayer like that!

Use your prayer journal and prayer time this week to seek ways in which you can be obedient to God.

Lord Jesus, You have shown me Your love through Your obedience to the Father. Give me the strength and desire to answer "Yes, Lord" when You call.

God, You know my limits and weaknesses; You know every part of me. Help me to be obedient to Your will.

DAY 6: *Reflections*

In this week's study you have learned the importance of being obedient to God's plan and what He asks you to do. Obedience to God's will leads to answered prayer. Being obedient to God's will requires that you know His Word, so memorizing Scripture will help you to be obedient. Last week you learned to worship, confess, thank and petition God in prayer—memorizing and using Scripture as you pray helps you to do these things. There are still three other important reasons for memorizing Scripture:

1. It helps you handle difficult situations.
2. It helps you overcome temptation.
3. It gives you direction and guidance in your daily actions.

As you read and study the Bible, write down verses that have special meaning or may be of particular help to you. Choose one or two verses to memorize each week. As you memorize new verses, review the old ones until they become a part of you. Using the verses as you pray gives them new meaning and power as you battle the strongholds in your life.

No matter what the situation or problem may be, God has an answer to be found in His Word. Search and memorize Scripture; then pray using the Word to set you free from the bondage of your strongholds.

Allow the following prayers from Beth Moore's book *Praying God's Word* to put you on the right track.

My Lord, hear me and answer me. My thoughts trouble me and I am distraught (see Psalm 55:2).

Lord, help me not to fear, for You are with me; I need not be dismayed, for You are my God. You will strengthen me and help me; You will uphold me with Your righteous right hand (see Isaiah 41:10).[1]

Lord of heaven and Earth, help me to be still and know You are God; You will be exalted among the nations. You will be exalted in the earth. You, Lord Almighty, are with me; the God of Jacob is my fortress (see Psalm 46:10,11).

DAY 7: *Reflections*

This week's memory verse gives clear instruction about obedience. Jesus says that whoever has His commands and obeys them is the one who loves Him. Do you love Him? Are you keeping His commands? Are you obeying His will?

These are hard questions for Christians to answer. Saying you love Him is easy, but showing it is difficult. By studying God's Word diligently, you find peace, comfort and strength to obey. Being obedient may bring pain or discomfort in the beginning, but the end result is the "peace of God, which transcends all understanding" (Philippians 4:7). Are you ready for God's will to be done in your life through obedience to Him? If you are, then He will answer your prayers.

Memorizing Scripture helps you to personalize verses, gives you ownership of the truth and guides you to obedience. One problem with Scripture memory is remembering the reference. Each time you say the verse, begin and end with the reference to help you glue it in your mind.

The music CD that accompanies this Bible study is an excellent resource to help you memorize Scripture. Listen to it in your car or at home while you're doing chores or exercising. Through this practice, the Holy Spirit will be able to bring to your mind the truths you need in times of difficulty.

As you complete this third week of Bible study, repeat the memory verse. Each time you use the verse, God plants it more firmly in your mind and heart.

Oh Lord, in You my heart rejoices for I trust Your holy name. May your unfailing love rest upon me, O Lord, as I put my hope in You (see Psalm 33:21,22).

Lord, I will praise You with an upright heart as I learn Your righteous laws. I will obey Your decrees for I know You will not utterly forsake me (see Psalm 119:7,8).

Lord God, I pray that Your love may abound in me more and more with knowledge and depth of insight so that I will know what is best and that I may be pure and blameless, filled with the fruit of righteousness that comes through Jesus Christ (see Philippians 1:9,11).

Heavenly Father, You have said that if I hear your commands and obey them, I show my love for You and that because You love me, Your Father will love me. Help me to be obedient and prove my love for You (see John 14:21).

Note
Beth Moore, *Praying God's Word* (Nashville, TN: Broadman and Holman, 2000), pp. 254, 255, 321.

GROUP PRAYER REQUESTS   TODAY'S DATE: 4/11/03

NAME	REQUEST	RESULTS

EXCUSES, EXCUSES

Week Four

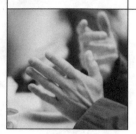

MEMORY VERSE
*You know my folly, O God;
my guilt is not hidden from you.*
Psalm 69:5

Excuses. We all make them. So what is an excuse? An excuse is a lie disguised as a reason.

Take away our excuses, and we're forced to assume personal responsibility for our actions. Take away our excuses, and we have no place to hide. We can only stand and stare in the mirror, knowing we must deal with ourselves.

In this week's study, you'll have the chance to deal honestly with your excuses. You'll discover that real progress in life begins when you stop making excuses and you start being honest with yourself and with God.

DAY 1: *So Many Choices*

Why do we make excuses? Is it because we don't want to assume responsibility for our poor choices? Every day we must make choices and some of them are not the best choices. Why do we make wrong choices? Because we might believe that we are making good ones. Sometimes we might make choices on the spur of the moment without thinking the situation through. Other times we make wrong choices because we have taken the poor advice of another person.

In order to understand why we make wrong choices, let's look at what happened "in the beginning." The first wrong choice occurred in the Garden of Eden with Adam and Eve's decision to disobey God. God created Adam and Eve; then He gave them free will to make choices. Theirs was the most costly choice ever made. Genesis 2:16,17 describes the choice Adam and Eve had.

>> What was God's command?

>> What would be the consequence of making the wrong choice?

>> In Genesis 3:1, how did Satan's question create doubt concerning what God said?

>> How did Satan contradict God in verse 4?

Adam and Eve believed Satan's lie. Even though God had filled the world with all the good things Adam and Eve needed, they believed Satan and focused on the one thing they were told they could not have. God gives us everything we need in the world today, including healthy foods and other healthy options. Unfortunately, there are also some unhealthy things in this world. We have choices to make and Satan loves to tempt us, contradicting what God says. Don't believe Satan.

>> Why do you think God gave Adam and Eve choices?

>> Why does God give you choices to make concerning your health and lifestyle?

You have the freedom to make choices in your life—either good or bad ones. God will help you make the right choices so that His work can be accomplished in your life. Instead of listening to Satan's lies, look to God for truth.

⟱ According to John 8:31,32, what will God's truth do in your life?

Commit yourself to live in God's truth. Refuse to listen to Satan's lies. Be honest with yourself and God and His truth will set you free.

> Dear Lord, I thank You for giving me choices to make in my life, and I pray for Your guidance in making the right choices.
>   Father, I pray for Your strength to help me resist and flee Satan when he lies to me.

DAY 2: *Discovering Who is Responsible*

Why did God include the tree of the knowledge of good and evil in the Garden of Eden? He knew what would happen. He could have created a world without choices. He could have told Adam and Eve, "Here's a wonderful garden filled with everything you need. By the way, I don't want you to eat the fruit of that tree over there. But don't worry, I've created you in such a way that you won't want that fruit anyway." Wouldn't this be the perfect plan—people engineered in such a way that they could only make right choices?

In a hypothetical garden in which Adam and Eve could not, by God's design, desire to eat the forbidden fruit, who would ultimately be responsible for their actions?

☐ God would be responsible.
☐ God would be responsible.
☐ God would be responsible.

Congratulations! You've selected the correct answer. Do you feel a sense of accomplishment? Do you get the point? Without the opportunity to choose the right or wrong answer, there is no victory in choosing the correct one.

The Old Testament is full of examples of how God gave choices in many situations. Genesis 22:1-18 tells of Abraham's willingness to obey God's command by sacrificing his son, Isaac.

➤ According to Genesis 22:12-18, what was the result of Abraham's choosing to obey God?

➤ Joshua 24:14,15 tells of someone who made a choice for God. Who is speaking and what was the choice he made?

Each of these leaders of the Old Testament took responsibility for his actions and chose to obey and serve God. When right choices are made, rewards and blessings result. Wrong choices lead to suffering and punishment. Everyone must make the ultimate choice: to love and obey God *or* to reject and disobey Him.

Thank God for making it possible for you to make choices and for giving you the guidance and wisdom to make right choices. Have you made the choice to love Him?

Heavenly Father, I thank You for loving me and giving me the choice to love You.

Precious Lord and Savior, I am responsible for making the right choices. Guide me and instruct me in the way I should go.

DAY 3: *Following Directions*

God clearly communicated His rules to Adam and Eve, but they chose to disobey. God's commands established the boundaries for proper actions, and He warned them of the consequences of stepping outside the boundaries. Armed with God's commands and warnings, Adam and Eve had all they needed to make the right choice.

➣ Psalm 1:1-3 describes the results of obeying God. What is the delight of the person who walks with God?

➣ Summarize the blessing in your own words.

➣ In Titus 2:11,12, what does the grace of God teach us to do?

When you delight in God's Word, you will experience the life pictured in Psalm 1. As you meditate on God's law day and night, you will learn how to resist the false statements and half truths of those who reject God. The obedient Christian life is characterized by vitality, energy and purpose.

In the Old Testament there are many instances in which people chose to disobey God. When they chose to disobey, God rained down punishment time and time again. The Israelites had short memories and continued to make wrong choices; yet several individuals chose to follow God and obey His plans and direction. One such man was Daniel.

☙ Read Daniel 1. What choice did Daniel make that is recorded in verse 8 and what was the result, according to verse 9?

☙ According to verse 17, how did God reward Daniel and his three friends for their obedience?

Judges 7 is the account of a warrior named Gideon whom God chose to save Israel. Gideon made many excuses, but finally chose to follow God. He prepared to fight a battle with a large army, but God continued to instruct Gideon to make the army smaller and smaller. Finally, he had only 300 soldiers left to fight the mighty army of the Midianites. Yet each time Gideon did as he was instructed, he was blessed.

☙ According to Judges 7:19-22, what was the result of Gideon's obedience?

Throughout the Bible we are shown how to live in obedience to God's directions. Commit yourself to learning more about God's Word so that you can live according to His truth. He will help you make choices in life that will cause your life to prosper and flourish.

 Dear Lord, I know Your directions will lead me to a more abundant life. Thank you for loving me and giving me guidance.

Father God, help me to live my life in complete obedience to the directions You give me through Your Word.

DAY 4: _Not My Fault_

Strange, isn't it, that the first real choice in the world involved eating? It shouldn't surprise anyone that food also prompted the world's first excuses. What excuses have you heard others make for their indulgences in poor lifestyles?

- I don't have time to exercise.
- This problem runs in my family.
- I'm nervous, and I do this because it calms my nerves.
- I don't get enough sleep because I have too much to do at night.
- It's a medical problem.

Have you made any of these excuses? It's easy to find excuses for not doing what is right and to indulge in things that may harm your health. When it comes down to the bottom line, you must admit the truth. No one else is responsible for your actions.

Genesis 3:12,13 tells how Adam and Eve answered God after eating the forbidden fruit.

➤ What were their excuses?

Excuses—lies disguised as reasons. Adam's excuse was the most creative. Who was he actually blaming? Eve or God? Look at Genesis 3:12 and decide.

Adam, like so many others, didn't want to assume responsibility for his actions. Can't you hear Adam stammering and stuttering his excuse to God? "That woman is to blame—not me. Why did you put her in this garden anyway?" Eve joined Adam in dodging responsibility. She blamed the serpent.

➤ In Genesis 3:9, what question did God ask Adam?

➤ Why did God ask that question? Do you think He really didn't know where they were?

God doesn't lose things. Perhaps He wanted Adam and Eve to know that He knew what they had done and why they were trying to hide.

Are you trying to fool others with your excuses and rationalizations about your life? You may fool other people, and you may even fool yourself into believing your excuses. However, you will never fool God.

Satan is the father of lies. He twists what God says. He urges you to believe your own excuses. He baits and traps you with lies people love to believe. The following are examples of excuses Satan tries to trap you into believing:

- This really isn't that bad.
- It might hurt some people, but it won't hurt you.
- You deserve better than this.
- Don't expect God to look out for you. You're on your own.

If Satan can cause you to doubt something God has said, he can position you for a wrong choice. That's what he did with Eve. He planted doubt through a simple question: "Did God really say . . . ?" Don't let yourself fall for his lies. You will not progress in the Christian life until you accept responsibility for your own choices.

 Lord, I thank You for Your power to help me make better choices in the future.

Lord God, teach me Your truth so that I can be set free from Satan's trap.

DAY 5: *Being Honest with God*

God knows all you have ever done or will do. Go ahead and be honest with Him. If you've made wrong choices in the past, confess them. God will forgive you. If your wrong choices have created tough consequences, accept them. Then God can begin to work to transform both you and your consequences.

David knew that he couldn't hide his sins from God, but he ignored what he had done until confronted by the prophet Nathan. Faced with the reality of his sin, David went to the Lord.

≫ In Psalm 69:5, what was David's realization?

≫ What does this verse mean to you?

≫ Psalm 51 is another prayer of David's in which he decided to be honest with God. What was David's confession in verses 3 and 4?

≫ What was his request in verses 10-12?

≫ What is the sacrifice that God wants, according to verse 17?

Excuses are jail bars that trap you and keep you from living a responsible life. You cannot make the changes you need to make, and God cannot work in you until you are honest with Him and confess your sins.

Break free from excuses and dishonesty with God. The following statements contain truths that will set you free. Check the statements you want to make part of your life as you leave the entrapment of excuses and embrace honesty.

- ☐ God knows everything about me and still loves me. I can be honest with Him.
- ☐ When I make wrong choices, I admit my sins and God forgives me.
- ☐ When my wrong choices create tough circumstances, I trust God to give me strength to work through them.
- ☐ I know I'm not perfect, but I am loved. God loves me just as I am. God loves me too much to allow me to stay where I am. God isn't finished with me yet.
- ☐ Satan may tempt me, but he cannot force me to make wrong choices. I can resist him. I choose to resist him through God's power.
- ☐ Sure, I've made some wrong choices in the past. God has forgiven my past. I've chosen to make God first place in my life and as a result of His power in my life, I have a great future.

When you recognize the fact that Satan will tempt you to make wrong choices, you can also know that God will help you to make right choices. Keep your eyes focused on Jesus and what He has promised to do for you. Satan will turn away each time you resist him, but he won't give up.

 Lord, help me to repel the father of lies.

God, You know my sins; my guilt cannot be hidden from You. Forgive my weaknesses and restore my joy.

DAY 6: *Reflections*

In this week's study you have learned about the excuses that we make for disobeying God. It's human nature to become defensive and make excuses or rationalize when confronted with the results of wrong choices.

Take away those excuses and the only ones left to assume responsibility for our wrong choices are ourselves.

The key to making good decisions and right choices is to keep your eyes focused on Jesus and the Word of God. This is another reason why memorizing Scripture becomes so important. When God's Word is imprinted on your heart and soul, the Holy Spirit recalls them for you when you need help. In addition, God's Word can help you give support to others who have choices to make. This is important in your First Place group as you encourage and support one another.

God's will for you is to believe in His Son, feed on His Word and live obediently. Feeding on His Word gives you the strength and stamina to fight the good fight against Satan just as Jesus did in the wilderness. When you study and memorize Scripture, you will always have His Word with you.

Pray sincerely, believing His Word and using His Name as you pray this week. Remember the words of Jesus: "Therefore I tell you, whatever you ask for in prayer, believe that you have received it, and it will be yours" (Mark 11:24). Claim God's promises in your prayer time and use His Word as you pray.

Father God, fill me with the fruit of righteousness that comes through Jesus Christ that I might give You all the glory and praise (see Philippians 1:11).

Lord, keep me from making excuses. Help me to serve only You. For You have promised to always be with me, to hold me by my right hand, to guide me with Your counsel and then to take me to glory (see Psalm 73:23,24).

Merciful God, hear my prayer. I confess my sin to You for You have promised to forgive my wickedness and remember my sins no more (see Jeremiah 31:34).

DAY 7: *Reflections*

The memory verse for this week reminds you that God knows your heart. He knows your sins. You cannot hide your guilt from Him, just as Adam and Eve in the Garden couldn't hide from God. Just as He gave Adam and

Eve choices, He gives you choices. You make choices about what to wear, what to eat, how to respond to people, what to do on the job, how to spend your time—the list is endless.

Many of your choices are automatic. How earnestly do you seek God's help in making choices? He's interested in everything that you do. He gives you the directions for living your life in Him. Read His Word and follow His directions.

Sometimes we can't make wrong choices right, as was the case with Adam and Eve. We must bear the consequences of our actions, but God does forgive us when we come to Him with repentant hearts. Perhaps God was more disappointed in Adam and Eve than He was angry. Their sin, and consequently our sin, led to the greatest sacrifice ever made—the death of God's own Son, Jesus Christ.

God has given us His Word to help us know how to make right choices. When you pray, use God's Word sincerely with true repentance, meaning what you say. Avoid merely saying the words—understand and mean the words with all your heart.

As you complete this week of Bible study, repeat the memory verse. Practice it often, and listen to the CD provided with this study. Each time you use the verse, God will plant this Scripture more firmly in your mind and heart.

 Lord God, help me to keep up my courage and my faith in You that things will happen just as You have said (see Acts 27:25).

Mighty God, help me to understand that I've been called by You to live by faith and not by sight. Strengthen my spiritual vision, Lord (see 2 Corinthians 5:7).

Heavenly Father, forgive my sin for You know my folly, and my guilt cannot be hidden from you (see Psalm 69:5).

GROUP PRAYER REQUESTS TODAY'S DATE:_____

NAME	REQUEST	RESULTS

GOOD NEWS ABOUT TEMPTATION

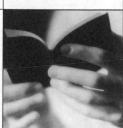

MEMORY VERSE

No temptation has seized you except what is common
to man. And God is faithful; he will not let you be tempted
beyond what you can bear. But when you are tempted, he will
also provide a way out so that you can stand up under it.
1 Corinthians 10:13

Quick. Name seven good things about temptation. Could you think of seven? Could you think of any? For most people, it's hard to think of anything good about temptation.

In this week's study, you'll discover some incredibly good news about temptation. As a result of what you learn, you'll be ready the next time sin entices you. In this week's study, you'll find seven (at least!) good things about temptation.

DAY 1: *The Same Old Story*

Here's the first good news about temptation, found in 1 Corinthians 10:13: "No temptation has seized you except what is common to man." When you're tempted to do something, say something or eat something you know you shouldn't, do you ever feel you're the only person in the world battling that temptation?

➤ Describe how you feel when tempted.

You can find comfort in the midst of temptation if you think about statements such as:

- Lots of people know what I'm feeling in this situation.
- I'm not the first, nor the last, to experience this temptation.
- Others have faced this temptation without giving in to it.

➤ Does it make you feel any better to know you are not alone in facing your temptation? Why or why not?

The first part of 1 Corinthians 10:13 describes temptation as strong, even aggressive. Temptation lurks like a mugger on a dark street. It lunges at you. It seizes you—it holds on and refuses to turn you loose. But James 1:13 states that you'll never have to worry about temptation coming from our loving God.

➤ What is the source of your temptation? And how does this make you feel?

➤ James 1:14,15 describes the face of this mugger known as Temptation. What actually seizes you when you are tempted?

God doesn't tempt you. Most people don't like to admit it, but their own evil desires seize them. Temptation begins in your fleshly desires. Then Satan knows how to step in to further tempt you. However, once you know the source of the temptation, you can attack it and defeat it.

The temptations facing you right now are nothing new. Others have faced them and conquered them. God can transform the evil desires in your heart if you ask Him to reveal them to you. Don't wait for temptation to seize you—go on the offensive through God's power in prayer.

Dear Lord, reveal my evil desires and give me the power to overcome them through Your precious name.

Father, forgive my sins and make me a new creature in You.

DAY 2: *Even When We Aren't Faithful*

We are constantly battling temptation in our lives. How can we fight? How can we win?

➤ Reread 1 Corinthians 10:13 to find how to win. What word does this passage use to describe God? What does this mean to you?

➤ In Yellowstone National Park is a geyser named Old Faithful. Why do you think people gave the geyser this name?

Undoubtedly, it took a number of years for people to associate the name Old Faithful with one particular geyser. Over time, however, it demonstrated such consistency that people assumed it would act in a predictable way.

One of the central principles of the Christian life is that God is trustworthy. Initially, you can affirm God's faithfulness intellectually, but through your experiences with Him, you will begin to affirm God's faithfulness personally and emotionally. You can declare, "I've been through many things in my life, and God has never let me down. He has been faithful."

➤ What has happened, or what would have to happen, to cause you to declare with conviction that God is faithful in times of temptation?

How is God described in Psalm 73:26? How can this description give you confidence in God?

What is the promise in Romans 6:14 and how does this promise encourage you?

God promised to be faithful to you in times of temptation. When temptation comes, see if God keeps His Word and helps you withstand the temptation. Each time He does—and He will—your personal understanding of God's faithfulness will grow. In time, you'll be able to say with passion and conviction, "Even when I'm tempted, God is faithful to me."

Revelation 21:7 tells of the reward for those who resist the temptations of the world. What is the promise of this verse?

God is faithful and will teach you more about His faithfulness as you read His Word.

Heavenly Father, I thank You for being faithful even when I am unfaithful.

Precious Lord and Savior, You promised to deliver me from my sins and make a way of escape when I am tempted. Help me to believe and trust You and Your Word.

DAY 3: *Setting the Limits*

When you are tempted, have you ever made statements such as these?

- I couldn't help myself, the temptation was too strong.
- No one could have turned that down—especially not me.
- I wanted to stop, but I just lost control.

When you give in to temptation, you are more likely to believe you really had no choice. But 1 Corinthians 10:13 tells you the truth about temptation. God sets limits on temptation. That's more good news.

➤ Based on 1 Corinthians 10:13, what do you think God would say if you were to give in to temptation and offer the excuse "I just couldn't help myself"?

God never promised we would not be tempted. He never promised temptations would be easy to resist. He has, however, set limits on the degree to which we can be tempted. As a result, we can know that any temptation we experience can be overcome. God knows the level of temptation you can resist and expects you to resist.

➤ According to Ephesians 6:10,11, how are you to prepare for the devil's schemes?

➤ James 1:12 explains the rewards of resisting temptation. What is the result when you face your trials and stand the test?

Stand firm in God's power. The memory verse reminds you that God is faithful. When you find yourself in the midst of strong temptation, remember the words of 1 Corinthians 10:13—repeat them now.

 Dear Lord, You apparently think I can bear stronger temptation than I would have thought possible. With Your help, I will resist.

Father God, help me to put on the full armor so that when I am tempted, I can stand my ground and resist.

DAY 4: *Preparing for What's Coming*

God warns that temptation is coming. Expect temptation. First Corinthians 10:13 says, "but *when* you are tempted" (emphasis added).

➤ If you know you are going to be in a situation in which you will be tempted by others, what steps can you take to prepare for battle before temptation begins?

➤ According to John 8:32, why is truth important for you?

➤ Remind yourself of God's truth and focus on the truths found in the memory verse. List three truths about temptation found in 1 Corinthians 10:13.

1.

2.

3.

You are most vulnerable to temptation when it surprises you. However, since you know you will be tempted every day, you should be constantly prepared. Each day attempt to anticipate the temptations you will face. Plan how you will fight and defeat them.

➤ How can you plan for the possible temptations that will come into your life during the day?

Temptation presses down on your life. When you ask God to remove the temptation, He has another plan: Stand up under it. Fighting temptation may feel like holding a heavy weight above your head. You will struggle under the burden.

➤ Matthew 4:1-11 describes how Jesus handled temptation in a particular situation in His life. How long had Jesus gone without food?

➤ Why do you think Satan's first temptation was related to the physical?

➤ What did Jesus do to resist Satan's temptation?

Jesus faced temptation. He battled. He won. Every time Satan enticed Him, Jesus countered with God's Word. He wants you to win too and He will provide what you need to resist. God wants you to be mature and complete, lacking nothing. Temptation is one of the trials that will help you to mature and grow strong in faith.

➤ According to James 1:2-4, why does God tell you to consider times of testing, trial and temptation as pure joy?

➤ How would you apply the truth of these verses in time of temptation so you could be joyful in the midst of difficulties?

Obviously, God knows you do not enjoy trials. He expects you to look beyond the trials to the positive changes trials produce. God wants you to see the connection between the trials you face with the character and maturity developing in you.

Lord, make me wise in dealing with my temptations. Help me to anticipate and then resist those that come my way.

Lord God, I know You do not tempt me. Temptation comes from Satan and my own evil desires. Help me to follow Your guidance in every area of my life.

DAY 5: *The Exit in Temptation Alley*

Picture temptation as a long dark alley. You turn a corner and enter the alley unexpectedly. You panic. You walk faster and faster. At the end of Temptation Alley stands sin. Sin waits for you, hoping temptation brings you to him. Each step brings you closer. What can you do? Are you trapped? Is there no way out?

➤ First Corinthians 10:13 is the good news, showing your escape from Temptation Alley! What does God say He will do for you?

Picture yourself running down that long, dark alley. Suddenly you notice doorways to your right and left. Above one door glows a green exit sign. God has promised to provide your exit out of Temptation Alley.

Jesus used one of those exits when He was tempted in the wilderness. Each time Satan offered another temptation, Jesus stood up to him and won.

➤ Luke 4:1-12 gives an account of Jesus' encounter with Satan's temptation. How can you use this strategy in your personal battle with temptation?

➤ Think back to an occasion when you were faced with a strong temptation but managed to resist. What exit did you use?

➤ Imagine yourself in a temptation sneak attack. Friends give you a surprise party. Spread out on the table are your favorites: snack foods, sweets and desserts. How could you use 1 Corinthians 10:13 to stand up under the pressure of this temptation?

God promised to provide an exit. He has not, however, promised to provide multiple opportunities for exiting Temptation Alley. Learn to look for God's exit. As soon as you realize you are facing temptation, your reflex response should be to pray to find God's exit immediately. He has promised to answer that prayer.

➤ Ephesians 6:10,11 describes how to prepare for the devil's schemes. What are we to do? What will be the result when we prepare?

Lord, thank You for the exit sign you provide. Help me to recognize Your exit early and then to take it quickly.

Father God, thank You for providing the power to stand firm under the pressures of temptation. Help me to remember to not rely on my puny weapons but to put on Your armor each day.

DAY 6: *Reflections*

In this week's study you have learned about the importance of facing temptation with the help of the Lord. He will give you a way of escape. He will help you to stand strong under pressure, and He never allows you to be tempted beyond your strength.

The most dangerous consequence of giving in to temptations is that, if not checked, they lead to strongholds. Greed, lying, lust, deceitfulness, gambling, alcohol, drugs, gluttony, uncontrolled temper, prejudice, selfishness, jealousy, an uncaring heart and pride can become strongholds that take over your life and destroy it. God can forgive you and release you from these strongholds. However, once they are forgiven and you put them out of your life, Satan calls them up and tries to entice you into his ways once again. That's when God's Word becomes the exit, the escape for you.

The key to resisting temptation is the same you would use in making choices—keep your eyes focused on Jesus. Let the words that come from your mouth and the thoughts of your mind be centered on Him. Reading His Word daily and committing it to memory assures that you will have His Words ready to help you in any situation. Jesus battled Satan with God's truth. You must do the same. Each verse you memorize in First Place provides another weapon in your battle against temptation.

Put on the whole armor of God. Know the weapons He has provided for you. Read and memorize Ephesians 6:10-18. Be strong in the Lord and His mighty power, and you will stand firm when Satan comes your way. Be prepared for Satan and he won't be able to attack you unaware.

Father God, Your Word says I am to love the Lord and hate evil, for You will guard the life of Your faithful servant and deliver me from the hand of the wicked. Deliver me, O God, from the lies of Satan (see Psalm 97:10).

Lord, help me to have no fear of disaster or ruin that comes to the wicked, for You are my confidence and will keep my foot from being trapped (see Proverbs 3:25,26).

Merciful God, You are my hiding place. You will protect me from trouble and surround me with songs of deliverance (see Psalm 32:7).

DAY 7: *Reflections*

This week's memory verse shows that God provides for you when you are tempted. He knows that everyone is subject to temptation, so He makes provision for His children just as loving parents make provision to keep their children safe.

God is committed to building your character and transforming you into the image of Christ. The transformation isn't quick and easy. He wants you to be mature and complete, lacking nothing. You will face trials and temptations. Remember God's promise in Deuteronomy 30:11: He will not command you to do anything that is too difficult or beyond your reach. Remind yourself of this as you face the trials and temptations that come into your life.

Read the following statements as well as the verse that goes with each one. Select several or all of them to memorize and use when you are tempted.

- The temptations I face are not new nor am I the only one tempted (see Romans 3:23).
- God is faithful; I can count on Him (see 1 Thessalonians 3:3).
- God will not allow me to face temptation I cannot resist (see Psalm 18:39).
- Since I know temptation is coming, I can be prepared to resist (see 1 Peter 1:13).
- When I am tempted, God provides a way out (see 1 Corinthians 10:13).
- I can stand up under the pressure of temptation (see Romans 6:14).
- God uses pressure in my life to build character (see James 1:2-4).

Charles Stanley, in his book *In Touch with God*, writes, "God's ultimate desire for us is not that we should be delivered from being tempted, but that we should be delivered through temptation."[1] God knows what you can bear and will not allow you to be tempted beyond your limits, and He will provide the way out of every situation that produces temptation for you.

Remind yourself to use the Scripture memory CD while exercising, doing chores, driving or during work breaks. Through memorization, the Holy Spirit will be able to show you the truths you need for whatever comes into your life.

As you complete this week of Bible study, repeat the memory verse. Each time you use the verse, God plants this Scripture more firmly in your mind and heart. With confidence in God's provision, you will resist the temptations that come.

Pray today for God's protection in times of temptation. Put on His whole armor and stand fast in your faith.

Father, You taught us to pray and ask not to be led into temptation but to be delivered from evil, for Yours is the kingdom and the power and the glory forever. Deliver me from the evil one and all his lies, so I may live with You eternally (see Matthew 6:13).

Mighty God, You instructed me not to love the world or the things in the world, for if I love the world, the love of the Father is not in me. Everything that tempts me from the world—the lust of the flesh, the lust of the eyes and the pride of life—is not of You, O Father. Help me to love You and only You, and dwell in me so that I may not sin (see 1 John 2:15,16)

Father God, help me to get rid of all immoral filth and the evil that is so prevalent, and help me to humbly accept the Word planted in me which can save me (see James 1:21).

O Lord, help me to know the truth, for it is the truth that sets me free (see John 8:32).

Heavenly Father, I know Your Word and trust You because You have told me that there is no temptation that comes that is not common to all people and that You will not allow me to be tempted with anything I cannot bear. I claim Your promise of provision for a way out so that I can stand firm and strong under it (see 1 Corinthians 10:13).

Note
Charles Stanley, *In Touch with God* (Nashville, TN: Thomas Nelson Inc., 1997), p. 77.

GROUP PRAYER REQUESTS   TODAY'S DATE:_____

NAME	REQUEST	RESULTS

TRUE SATISFACTION

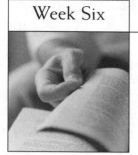

MEMORY VERSE
Man does not live on bread alone,
but on every word that comes from the mouth of God.
Matthew 4:4

On one occasion, a reporter asked billionaire J. Paul Getty, "How much money is enough?" Mr. Getty replied, "Just a little bit more." We could change the question to "How much food is enough?" and all too often the answer would be "Just a little bit more."

Physical desires can become demanding, controlling our lives like a spoiled two-year-old. Appease those initial desires with instant self-indulgence, and the demands only intensify. Christ died to free us from sin, from compulsion, from a life out of control. How tragic if we fail to use Christ's power to break the destructive desires in our lives.

In this week's study, you'll learn about God's plan for true satisfaction. Your success in the First Place program depends on it.

DAY 1: *Spiritual Food Required*

In the Beatitudes Jesus tells Christians how to find satisfaction in life. Each one begins with the word "blessed." You could substitute the word "blessed" with the phrase "Oh, the wonderful joy of." You will find the Beatitudes in Matthew 5:3-10.

➤ According to Matthew 5:6, what should you seek?

➤ With what intensity should you seek it?

≫ What will be the result of your search?

Righteousness is a major theme of the Bible. Like a diamond, the word "righteousness" has many facets. For now, think of righteousness as having a right standing with God. When you want a right relationship with God more than you want anything else in life, you will be satisfied.

≫ Romans 1:17 states the basis of your righteousness before God. Rewrite this verse in your own words.

God called you to a life of faith. Through faith, you trust that you can have a right standing with God because Jesus Christ died for you. If God had not paid for your sins through the Cross, you could never experience His love. Your sin would demand God's judgment and would keep you separated from Him.

≫ When people have a problem in their relationship with God, how does that compound the problems they have in the others areas of their lives?

Until our relationship with God is right, our lives won't be right. God designed you so He could live in you through His Holy Spirit. He never intended for you to face the demands of life and the enticement of temptation without His power. We each have a fundamental spiritual need for God, and we can't experience lasting satisfaction in our lives until we establish our relationship with God through Jesus Christ.

Ephesians 2:4-10 contains wonderful truth about salvation: You are precious to God, and He has provided the way for you to have a special relationship with Him.

➤ What do these verses tell you about your relationship with God?

➤ What wonderful news: God has *given* you salvation through His Son, Jesus Christ! In Romans 12:1, Paul described what our response needs to be. Rewrite this verse in your own words.

➤ Check the following statements if they are true about you. If you cannot check every box, talk with your pastor or a Christian friend about your uncertainty.

  ☐ I have begun a relationship with Jesus Christ.
  ☐ I am now righteous in God's eyes because of my faith in Christ.
  ☐ I have right standing with God because of Jesus' death on the cross.
  ☐ I am sure I am a Christian.

Dear Lord, help me grow in my relationship with You, because You have loved me and sent the Holy Spirit to live in me.

 Father, thank You for loving me and forgiving my sins. Teach me Your ways and guide me in all that I do as I work toward my goal.

DAY 2: *More to Life Than Our Desires*

Jesus faced a time of intense temptation at the beginning of His ministry. After Jesus had fasted for 40 days, Satan urged Him to set aside the Father's plan for His life and instead indulge His physical and emotional needs. Food, wealth, power, popular acclaim—Satan offered immediate gratification of these desires, but Jesus rejected every one.

➤ Matthew 4:1-4 describes how Satan tempted Jesus in the wilderness. When he tempted Jesus by saying, "Tell these stones to become bread," what was Jesus' response?

➤ What two important ideas are contained in Jesus' response?

1.

2.

➤ What do you think Jesus meant by His first statement about living on bread alone? How can this apply to your life?

➤ What do you think Jesus meant by living on "every word that comes from the mouth of God" (v.4)? How does this apply to your life?

In this passage Jesus affirmed that spiritual matters are more important than physical matters. He didn't deny the importance of physical needs, but through His extended time of fasting He modeled that physical needs pale in comparison to living by God's Word. Food, power and popular acclaim have their place, but compared to knowing God, they are nothing. Jesus was content and satisfied with what His Father provided.

➤ Another person in the New Testament who learned to be content in any situation was Paul. Rewrite Philippians 4:11-13 in your own words.

➤ In Philippians 4:19, Paul reveals more of the secret to contentment. What does this verse tell you about the abundance of God?

In Christ we find both satisfaction in life and the strength to meet life's demands. In Christ we find the abundant love that meets our emotional needs.

➤ According to Psalm 90:14, what will God do for us each morning?

➤ What was David's response to that love? Is it your response?

 Heavenly Father, I thank You for Your provision of spiritual food each day and for giving me Your love each day. Let me sing for joy and be glad in Your unfailing love.

Precious Lord and Savior, help me to be content in all circumstances and situations in my life and have faith to believe You will supply all my needs.

DAY 3: *The Bible—Spiritual Food*

On one occasion, the Old Testament prophet Ezekiel received a vision from God. In his vision, God gave him scrolls—comparable to our Bible today. The experience is described Ezekiel 3:1-3.

➤ Although you can't physically eat the Bible, how can you be filled to satisfaction with the Word of God?

➤ In Psalm 119:103, what response did the psalmist have to God's Word?

➤ What response do you usually have to God's Word?

Many Christians want to make God's Word, the Bible, an integral part of their lives, but they don't know how to start. The acrostic H-E-A-R-T can help you feast on God's Word. Read the following verses that make up this acrostic:

H   reminds me to **hear** God's Word.
       (See Romans 10:17.)

E   reminds me to **examine** (or read) God's Word.
       (See Revelation 1:3.)

A   reminds me to **analyze** (or study) God's Word.
       (See 2 Timothy 2:15.)

R   reminds me to **remember** (or memorize) God's Word.
       (See Psalm 119:11.)

T   reminds me to **think about** (or meditate on) God's Word.
       (See Psalm 1:2,3.)

➤ Why is doing as these verses suggest so important to you as a Christian (see Psalm 119:11)?

As you continue to give Christ first place in your life, God will place His Word in your H-E-A-R-T and will nourish you spiritually. He will meet your deep spiritual needs as no one and nothing else can, and you will find success in reaching your goals.

Dear Lord, let me hide Your Word in my heart so that I will be filled with the Words You speak to me.

Father God, Your Words are sweet to my taste and sweeter than honey to my mouth. Help me to eat and be filled daily.

DAY 4: *Doing God's Work Brings Satisfaction*

Jesus encountered a woman at a well in Samaria. The experience not only changed her life, but it taught Jesus' disciples an important spiritual principle.

➤ In John 4:4-15, what was the living water Jesus offered the Samaritan woman?

➤ What was the woman's response?

➤ Where were the disciples while Jesus talked with the woman?

➤ Continue by reading John 4:16-38. When the disciples returned, what did they urge Jesus to do (see verse 31)?

➤ How did Jesus respond to them in verse 32?

≫ The disciples thought someone had brought Jesus food, but what did Jesus tell them about the food He had?

≫ What did Jesus tell them to do?

Jesus taught His disciples that doing the Father's work was like eating spiritual food. Spiritual work satisfied Jesus so fully that physical food was less important to Him. The disciples were so focused on getting Jesus something to eat that they were missing the spiritual opportunities around them. Only when Jesus challenged them to open their eyes did they see the work God wanted them to do.

≫ According to John 4:39-42, what happened to the Samaritans in Sychar because Jesus took the time to speak to the woman at the well?

Jesus focused on spiritual needs and reaped a spiritual harvest. The disciples had focused on physical needs and would have missed the spiritual harvest had not Jesus challenged them to see the spiritual needs all around them and respond.

Because the Samaritans believed Jesus, they found satisfaction in the right place. Too often people look for satisfaction in the wrong places and are frustrated when the things of the world such as food, alcohol, drugs and sex can't satisfy their emotional and spiritual hunger. God warns us about looking for satisfaction in the wrong places.

≫ In your own words, describe the guidance found in Isaiah 55:2.

Accept the challenge to see the spiritual needs around you. As you seek to satisfy the needs of others through Jesus, He will satisfy your needs even more abundantly.

Lord, open my eyes so that I see the many opportunities for witnessing and sharing with others what You have done for me.

Lord God, give me the satisfaction and contentment I need to make my life what You would have it be, and fill me with the living water of eternal life.

DAY 5: *Jesus—Our Bread of Life*

You cannot be spiritually satisfied until you develop a close, personal relationship with Jesus Christ. That relationship becomes spiritual food for you, food that satisfies.

In the early stages of Jesus' ministry on Earth, crowds followed Him because He performed miracles; they were hoping that He was the military and political Messiah for whom they had waited—the one who would liberate them from their oppressor, Rome. We read in John 6:1-15 how Jesus miraculously fed a multitude, and how, as a result, the crowd tried to force Him to be their earthly king.

⇛ What were the disciples' concerns (see vv. 7-9)?

⇛ What did Jesus provide?

⇛ How did Jesus rebuke the crowd in John 6:26,27?

The crowd didn't want a relationship with Jesus; they wanted Jesus to meet their needs and entertain them. They didn't care about knowing Him or learning from Him; they sought Jesus to take care of their immediate needs.

➣ How did Jesus describe Himself in John 6:35?

➣ Why do you suppose He used this analogy?

Jesus described Himself as the "bread of life"—remember, He was teaching a group of people focused on physical hunger. Through word pictures such as "eats my flesh" and "drinks my blood" (John 6:54), Jesus challenged the people to make Him the focus of their lives, rather than physical food.

Imagine eating with Jesus as the 5,000 did, or even better, imagine having Jesus as a guest in your home, sitting at the table with you, enjoying a delicious meal. It can happen—at least spiritually.

➣ In Revelation 3:20, where is Jesus?

➣ What is He doing?

➣ What is Jesus waiting for?

Often this verse is used to tell non-Christians about Jesus and His desire to be part of their lives. In reality, the context indicates that this verse primarily applies to Christians. It is a challenge for believers to open wide the doors of their lives to Jesus. Notice He is not forcing His way in but gently knocking and waiting for us to respond by inviting Him in for fellowship.

 Lord, I know that only You can satisfy my emotional hunger. Become the bread of life in my life today.

God, I want to open the door into my life completely. I invite You to come in and take total control of my life.

DAY 6: *Reflections*

In this week's study, you have learned about the importance of looking to God to satisfy your emotional hunger. Too many people continue to hope that food, alcohol, drugs, sex or other physical temptations will satisfy that emotional hunger. The Bible warns of looking for satisfaction in the wrong places. Galatians 5:19-21 warns us concerning the acts of the sinful nature of humans. Those who live sinful lives cannot inherit the kingdom of God. The good news is that God sent the Holy Spirit to dwell in us and to help us in our battles against our sinful nature.

God's Word gives instruction in how to overcome the desires of the sinful nature. You may not be tempted by many of these sins, but no one is immune from all of them. If we think we're immune, we're being deceived by Satan into thinking that we're okay and don't need to worry. That is when we let our guard down, giving Satan his opportunity. Think about the acts of jealousy, anger, selfishness, selfish ambition, discord and dissension. Be careful that one of these emotional feelings or acts doesn't trip you up.

One solution is to commit God's Word to memory and use it often in your prayers and daily life. Follow the example set by Jesus Himself and quote Scripture when you feel your sinful nature trying to rear its head. Find verses that address your areas of greatest struggle and commit them to memory.

The most dangerous aspect of sin is not recognizing it for what it is, allowing it to become a stronghold. Pride is one sin that everyone must deal with. Pride will keep you from admitting when you are wrong or will prevent you from seeking help and/or forgiveness from others. Remember, God is the only one who is right all of the time! Repent from the sin of pride and He will forgive you. An overnight change could occur, but more than likely you will need to be vigilant and patient as God works in you over time.

Only in Christ can you find true satisfaction in life. Through Him you will find the strength to meet the demands of everyday life. The good news is that when you focus on Him and confess your sins to Him, the fruit of the Spirit—described in Galatians 5:22,23—will mature in your life.

Father God, I pray for the fruit of the Spirit—love, joy, peace, patience, kindness, goodness, faithfulness, gentleness and self-control—to become more evident in my life (see Galatians 5:22,23).

Lord, keep me from becoming weary in doing good so that I may, in the proper time, reap a harvest of blessings (see Galatians 6:9).

Merciful God, it is only because of Your great love for me and the richness of Your mercy that I was made alive in Christ even when I was dead in sin. Your grace has saved me (see Ephesians 2:4,5).

DAY 7: *Reflections*

This week's memory verse will remind you that God daily provides what you need through His Word. When physical desires become demanding and controlling, turn to the Bible for the comfort and spiritual food that will help you resist the physical desires that want to harm you. When you have Scripture memorized, you have His Word at your disposal anytime and anywhere.

At a church youth camp, the youth minister challenged the young people by taking away their Bibles for the week. The students were divided into family groups and told to pretend that they lived in a country

that did not allow Bibles or the worship of God. Each family was instructed to compile its own Bible from all they could remember from years of
Sunday School and Vacation Bible School. By the end of the week, all of
them were amazed at how much of the Bible they actually remembered
and wrote down in the proper order. All participants returned from that
camp with a new appreciation of not only the Bible but also the value of
memorizing Scripture.

You will probably never be in such a situation, but how would you do?
Could you quote and then write down enough verses to fill a book? What
a challenge! The more verses you memorize, the better equipped and
armed you are against the wiles of Satan.

God makes available the power to say no to sin and yes to Him. It is
up to you to use it. Remind yourself to use the Scripture memory CDs
while driving, exercising, doing chores or taking a break at work.

Repeat the memory verse. Each time you use the verse God will plant
this Scripture more firmly in your mind and heart. Through confidence in
God's provision you will be better able to resist the temptations that come
into your life.

 Father, help me to be both filled and hungry, to both abound
and suffer need because I know that true contentment comes
only from You and that I can do all things through Jesus, Your
Son, who strengthens me (see Philippians 4:12,13).

Mighty God, You have promised that if I endure, I shall
also reign with You. If I deny You, You will deny me. Help
me to keep my eyes on You and testify to Your grace (see
2 Timothy 2:12).

Heavenly Father, feed me with Your Word, for You have
said that man does not live on bread alone but on every word
that comes from the mouth of God (see Matthew 4:4).

GROUP PRAYER REQUESTS TODAY'S DATE:_____

NAME	REQUEST	RESULTS

THE SECRET TO PLEASING GOD

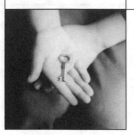

MEMORY VERSE

Do not conform any longer to the pattern of this world,
but be transformed by the renewing of your mind.
Then you will be able to test and approve what God's will is—
his good, pleasing and perfect will.

Romans 12:2

How do we know if Christ is first place in our lives? We don't know for sure until we have to make a choice. Inevitably, the time comes when we must decide between God's will and our own. Our choice reveals who is first place in our lives.

C. S. Lewis, in his book *The Great Divorce*, wrote that ultimately there are only two kinds of people in the world. First, there are those who say to God, "Thy will be done." Then there are those who stubbornly resist God's will; in the end, God says to them, "Thy will be done."[1]

In this week's study, you'll learn about God's will for your life. You'll discover that doing God's will is the best way to live and please God.

DAY 1: *The Privilege of Doing God's Will*

"God's will for your life": What is your initial impression of this phrase?

- ☐ God's will for my life would include everything I hate.
- ☐ God's will would be fine, but how can I discover it?
- ☐ God's will for my life is wonderful. I'm excited about it.

Many would check the first box. They fear God's will, convinced that He plans to make them miserable. Others would check the second box. They don't know how to know God's will for their lives. The third box is the optimum choice. The Bible clearly teaches that God's will for us is wonderful!

➤ List the characteristics found in Romans 12:2 that describe God's will for our lives.

1.

2.

3.

If you were offered something described as "good, pleasing and perfect," you would be excited to receive it, wouldn't you? That's exactly how you should feel about God's will. Following God's will in your life is your privilege. Nothing you can imagine could surpass God's plan for you.

➤ Considering that the Bible says God's will for your life is *good*, what would you anticipate in life if you did God's will?

➤ The Bible also says that God's will for you is *pleasing*. What would you anticipate in life if you did God's will?

➤ Since God's will for you is *perfect*, what would you anticipate in life if you did God's will?

If you do God's will, you can anticipate that you will do things that are *good*—morally good, never bad. You will do things that are *pleasing*—pleasing to God and ultimately satisfying to you. You will do things that are *perfect*—excellent, reaching the highest potential for your life.

Good, pleasing, perfect—this is God's will for your life. How can anything top that?

➤ According to Jeremiah 29:11-13, what is God's promise about His will for your life?

➤ How can you find God's will for your life?

 Dear Lord, thank You for the wonderful plans You have for my life. You are my hope and my future.

   Father, reveal Your perfect and divine will for my life so that I may joyfully follow Your plan and serve You.

DAY 2: *Ready to Do God's Will and Heed the Warnings*

You probably wish that your old nature could have dissolved the moment you became a Christian. Unfortunately, your old nature lives on. But as a Christian, you can relinquish the reins and offer control of your life to Christ living in you. God holds you accountable for that choice.

➤ You make choices in life and those choices are like seeds you sow. According to Galatians 6:8, what happens when you sow according to your sinful nature?

➤ How do wrong choices related to food fall into this category?

➤ What principles found in Romans 12:2 would help you discover God's will in making choices?

1.

2.

➤ What are some of the negative aspects of the world today that hinder your ability to know and do God's will in your life?

The most destructive path in this world is the focus on self. People become the center of their personal universe, living to please only themselves. As Christians we need to break the pattern of self-centeredness in our lives. You can't do God's will if you focus your energy on doing your own will. The only way to avoid wrong choices is to rely on God's strength to do His will in your life.

J. B. Phillips translated Romans 12:2 in this way: "Don't let the world around you squeeze you into its own mold, but let God remold your mind from within."

➤ List some attitudes you have right now that might need to be remolded.

You can't break out of the world's mold until you recognize you have been pressed into it. The more you know about God's Word, the easier it will be for you to recognize God's pattern and how it differs from the world's pattern.

➤ What new attitudes about your commitments would help you develop healthy habits?

Giving Christ first place in your life means living life according to His choices for you. This means making your choices based on what you know God would want you to do. You will know what God wants you to do from His Word.

> ➤ According to Matthew 7:21-23, how serious is the problem of continuing to live your own way?

Take God's warning seriously. Let Him transform your life by renewing your mind. He will help you break free from the self-centered ways of today's world.

 Heavenly Father, transform me by the renewing of my mind so that I will know what Your good, pleasing and perfect will is for my life.

Precious Lord and Savior, help me to break free from the desires of this world so that I can make choices in life that are pleasing and acceptable to You.

DAY 3: *Following Jesus' Example*

We can learn how to live as Christians by studying the life of Jesus. Two Scripture passages provide insight into Jesus' attitude about doing His heavenly Father's will. Jesus clearly understood His purpose on Earth. He also challenged His disciples to build their lives around that same purpose.

> ➤ According to John 6:38, what was Jesus' purpose for coming down from heaven?

> ➤ What challenge did Jesus give His disciples in John 15:10?

➤ What did Jesus mean in John 5:30 when He said He could nothing by Himself?

Our life purpose as followers of Jesus Christ is to do His will on Earth as He did His Father's will while on Earth. A similar principle is found in John 15:5 where Jesus describes our inability to accomplish anything of spiritual significance apart from Him.

➤ What happens as a result of not remaining in Christ?

The secret of pleasing God is to discover God's will and do it. Most of the time you may think of God's will on a personal level. You want to know whom to marry, where to live, what career to pursue. God's will includes these and other areas; however, God's will for you includes your place in His overall plan. You must ask, "What is God's overarching plan for my life?"

➤ How does God instruct you to live your life?

➤ Personalize Philippians 2:13 so that the verses applies specifically to you.

➤ How does Colossians 3:23 apply to you as you endeavor to follow Jesus' example?

Jesus lived to please God. That was His life's purpose. Jesus only did what the Father gave Him the power to do. That was His self-imposed limitation. God wants you to live in the same way. You must clearly understand your life's purpose—to please Jesus. You must clearly understand your limitations—without Jesus you can do nothing. With those principles in place, you're ready to do God's will.

➣ According to 1 Thessalonians 1:3, how were the people of Thessalonica pleasing to God?

Dear Lord, I know that without You I can do nothing that is pleasing or right. Guide me, Lord, and give me the wisdom I need for today.

Father God, help me to obey the commands You give me so that I may live a life that is acceptable and have complete joy in serving You.

DAY 4: *Attitude Check*

Whom do you want to please? Doing God's will begins with a desire to please *Him*.

The apostle Paul lived to please Jesus Christ. In the following Scripture passages, look for attitudes that helped Paul—and will help you—please God.

➣ What are your goals in life?

➣ In 2 Corinthians 5:9, Paul explained his goal. What was it?

➤ What is your role in life?

➤ In Galatians 1:10, how did Paul describe his role?

➤ To whom are you accountable in life?

➤ In 1 Thessalonians 2:4, Paul described why he sought to please God. What did God test in Paul's life? What did he mean by God testing his heart?

➤ How do you determine your agenda in life?

➤ In 2 Timothy 2:4, to what did Paul compare his life as a disciple of Christ?

The people of Thessalonica lived their lives in a way pleasing to God, but they were not perfect. In Paul's letters to the Thessalonian church, he listed the problems the people were having, but he also listed the things they were doing right.

≫ After reading 1 Thessalonians 1:3, list the characteristics of the Christians in Thessalonica.

≫ What was the characteristic described in 1 Thessalonians 4:9,10?

≫ What else did Paul say about the Thessalonians in 2 Thessalonians 1:4?

≫ From the list of characteristics below, check those that you wish to develop in your own life.

☐ Work produced by faith and labor prompted by love
☐ Endurance inspired by hope in Jesus Christ
☐ Strong faith in God and love for others
☐ Faith that continues to grow
☐ Love that is increasing
☐ Perseverance and faith in times of persecution and trials

Make it your primary goal today to please God and live as His servant, seeking only to do His will. You are accountable to Him; open your heart to His inspection and await His orders, for He is your Commanding Officer.

Lord, let me live today to please only You and to seek Your will for my life.

Lord God, give me an attitude of love toward those with whom I come into contact. Open my heart and fill it with Your love.

DAY 5: Start with Thanksgiving

Is doing God's will optional? Can you choose between God's will and your own will as if either is acceptable to God? God's will is a blessing for your life. Be thankful that He provides a way out of sin and into His love.

➤ First Thessalonians 5:18 states one specific aspect of God's will for your life. What is that will?

Some people believe doing God's will is complicated. One way to begin doing His will is by simply learning to be thankful. Anyone can express thanks to God; He expects you to live thankfully.

➤ Notice God doesn't tell you to be thankful *for* all circumstances. You are to be thankful *in* all circumstances. What is the difference between the two?

A study of the life of the apostle Paul shows how he lived a life of thanksgiving. No matter what circumstances he faced—and he faced some tough ones!—Paul remained thankful for the spiritual blessings that were his in Christ.

➤ Match the spiritual blessings with the Scripture passages:

1. 1 Corinthians 15:57 ___ a. The opportunity for spiritual service

2. 2 Corinthians 9:15 ___ b. The victory we have in Jesus Christ

3. 1 Timothy 1:12 ___ c. God's indescribable gift to us

How much better your life is when you claim the victory you have in Jesus and give thanks for His indescribable gift to you. Before David was the king of Israel, as a young boy he was a shepherd in his father's fields. Many of the psalms are David's words of thanksgiving, most of which he wrote during the worst of circumstances.

⋙ How did David praise God in each of the following verses?

Psalm 34:1-3

Psalm 66:1,2

Psalm 118:1

Psalm 136:1,2

Psalm 138:1-3

⋙ List some of your own spiritual blessings for which you can praise God and be thankful, no matter what circumstances you face.

 Lord, I open my mouth to sing praises to You and to thank You for all Your many blessings in my life.

God, help me to be thankful and to praise Your name no matter what circumstances may surround me.

DAY 6: *Reflections*

In this week's study you have learned the secret of pleasing God. He wants to be first place in your life and to show He is first place you must do His will. Scripture teaches you about God's will for your life. His will is nothing to fear, and once you seek Him and learn what He has for you, you will be excited.

Bible study and Scripture memory are part of your commitments in the First Place program to teach you more about God's will for your life. Look back over some of the verses from this week's lesson. Many of them are verses you should memorize so they will come to you in times of need or in times of praise and thanksgiving. They will forever be a reminder of God's love for you.

In 2 Timothy 3:16,17, we read about the importance of the study of Scripture. Memorizing Scripture equips you for every good work and arms you with "the sword of the Spirit, which is the word of God" and prepares you to face any battle before you (Ephesians 6:17).

The solution then to pleasing God is simple: Commit yourself to finding God's will by committing His Word to memory and using it often in your prayers and daily life. Remember that only in Christ can you find true satisfaction in life.

 Father God, teach me, rebuke me, correct me through Your Word which You inspired and gave to me so that I may be fully equipped to do Your good work (see 2 Timothy 3:16,17).

Lord, keep me from doing Your work out of selfish ambition or vain conceit, but let me serve in humility and concern for others (see Philippians 2:3).

Lord Jesus, help me to put on my new self, created to be like God in true righteousness and holiness (see Ephesians 4:24).

DAY 7: *Reflections*

This week's memory verse gives specific instruction about living in this sinful world. Romans 12:2 teaches us how to please God: He wants us to be transformed into new creatures with renewed minds; then we will know His good, pleasing and perfect will.

As you daily read the Scriptures, you will come across verses that are meaningful to you. One suggestion is to set up a section in your journal to categorize Scriptures that you find helpful. Use categories such as God's Will, Facing Temptation, Giving Thanks, God's Promises or any others you find helpful. In the appropriate sections write the verses you find.

Then begin to memorize the verses and use them as you face day-to-day problems, choices or situations in your life.

Having appropriate Scripture at your fingertips (or on the tip of your tongue!) to use in any situation provides you with a defense stronger than anything the enemy can hurl at you. Memorized Scripture also allows you to spend time with Him even when you don't have a Bible available. Memorizing His Word and doing what it says are always pleasing to God.

As you complete this week's Bible study, repeat the memory verse. Each time you use the verse, God plants His Word a bit deeper in your mind and heart, enabling you to resist the temptations that come your way.

 Lord Jesus, I eagerly expect and hope that I will in no way be ashamed, but will have sufficient courage so that now as always Christ will be exalted in my body, whether by life or by death (see Philippians 1:20).

Father God, I am suffering, but I am not ashamed. For I know whom I have believed, and I am convinced that You are able to guard what I have entrusted to You for that day (see 2 Timothy 1:12).

Father God, thank You for granting me repentance and leading me to a knowledge of the truth! Thank You for bringing me to my senses so that I could escape from the trap of the devil, who had taken me captive to do his will (see 2 Timothy 2:25,26).

Dear Heavenly Father, help me to no longer conform to the pattern of this world, but transform me by the renewing of my mind. Then will I be able to test and approve what Your will is for me: good, pleasing and perfect (see Romans 12:2).

Note
1. C.S. Lewis, *The Great Divorce* (New York: Collier Books, 1984), n.p.

GROUP PRAYER REQUESTS TODAY'S DATE:_____

NAME	REQUEST	RESULTS

VALUE YOUR BODY

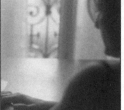

MEMORY VERSE

Do you not know that your body is a temple of the Holy
Spirit, who is in you, whom you have received from God?
You are not your own; you were bought at a price.
Therefore honor God with your body.
1 Corinthians 6:19,20

Don't ever take your body for granted. Your body is a precious resource.
Your body is important to God; therefore, it must be important to you. In
this week's study, we'll focus on seven reasons you should value your
body:

- Your body is the temple of God.
- God's Holy Spirit lives in you.
- God owns your body but entrusts it to you.
- God paid a high price for you.
- You can honor God with your body.
- You can dishonor God with your body.
- You can worship God with your body.

DAY 1: *Your Body—God's Temple*

Several verses in the New Testament refer to our bodies as God's temples
or as sacrifices to God. Read 1 Corinthians 3:16 for a vivid word picture
of your body as God's temple in which His Holy Spirit lives.

➤ What words or phrases do you associate with the word "temple"?

Many do not know much about temples. Some might associate temples with words such as "beauty" or "reverence" or "worship." When the Early Christians heard that they were the temples of the Holy Spirit, they understood the word picture. Temples were part of their lives and their history. As you learn more about temples, you will more fully understand what it means to be God's temple. Read the following passages that describe two characteristics of the Old Testament Temple:

➤ In 1 Kings 6:14-22,29-35 the structure of the Temple is described. What stands out to you in this description?

➤ According to 1 Kings 8:10-13 who dwelt in the Temple?

The Temple was a beautiful building. However, God's presence overshadowed the building's physical beauty.

➤ Based on these two descriptions, how do you feel about the fact that your body is the temple of the Holy Spirit?

Perhaps you don't feel like a beautiful temple right now. Most of us don't! However, when God filled the Temple with His presence, no one noticed the gold on the walls. So it is with your life. When God fills your life, you are a beautiful person. As God's light shines through your life, others will see Him in you.

In the Old Testament, the people of Israel worshiped in the beautiful Temple built by Solomon, but they didn't take care of it.

➤ According to 2 Kings 18:13-16, what did King Hezekiah do to the beauty of the Temple?

✎ According to 2 Kings 25:8,9, what finally happened to the Temple Solomon built?

✎ How tragic to think of the beautiful Temple in ruins. Do you ever feel like your temple is abused and in ruins? Describe your feelings about your temple.

The good news is that God can make something beautiful out of the ruins of your life. The Temple in Jerusalem was rebuilt from rubble. Ask God to make your life the beautiful spiritual temple He designed it to be.

✎ Read Hebrews 12:28, and then write a prayer expressing your love to God.

 Dear Lord, thank You for giving me a wonderful temple of worship in my body and help me to always honor You with all parts of my body.

Father, remove the strongholds from my life so that I may live a life pleasing to You, a life filled with Your Holy Spirit.

DAY 2: God's Address

Little children sometimes think God lives at church. One little boy thought the pastor kept God behind the curtains in the church baptistry! The Bible does reveal God's address. God lives in you and in every Christian.

➣ According to Habakkuk 2:20, where was God's presence in Old Testament times?

➣ According to 1 Corinthians 6:19, where does God live now?

Once you become a Christian, you know God's address. The incredible truth is that God lives in you. Your body has become His temple.

➣ Think back over the past week. To what degree have you been aware of God's presence in your life? Describe ways you sensed God's presence.

➣ There may be times you do not sense God's presence in your life, but Jesus has made a promise to us. What is the promise found in Matthew 28:20?

If Jesus were with you in His physical body and spent the entire day with you, how would His presence affect

🍎 Where you go?

🍎 What you do?

🍎 What you say?

🍎 What you eat?

Unfortunately, even with the best intentions, Christians might use their bodies to dishonor Christ. Through your body you can actually live as an enemy of the cross of Christ.

- According to Philippians 3:18,19, what characterizes the enemies of the Cross?

- In what ways can the things in your life, including eating habits, become your false gods?

Anything in life that begins to control you can become a god to you. Whatever controls you competes with the work that God wants to do in you. The truth is, if you are a Christian, God is with you every moment of every day. He knows what controls your life, and He can help you overcome anything that threatens to control you. Ask for His help so that what you do pleases and honors Him.

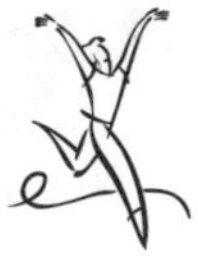

Heavenly Father, I know my body is Your temple. Help me to honor You in everything that I do every day.

Precious Lord and Savior, thank You for Your promise to be always with me, even to the end of the age.

DAY 3: *On Loan from God*

Have you ever borrowed something from a friend and forgotten to return it? Have you ever waited so long to return an item that you could no longer remember who had loaned it to you? God will not let us forget who owns our bodies! He states it clearly in His Word in this week's memory verse: "You are not your own."

Since your body belongs to God, not to you, you must ask, "What does God expect me to do with His property?"

Read the parable of the talents in Matthew 25:14-30 and answer the following:

↪ How did the master respond to the servants who used the money wisely?

↪ How did the master respond to the servant who used the money improperly?

We cannot, of course, hide anything from God. God knows every-thing we do. Since your body belongs to God and it has been entrusted to you by Him, what do you think He expects you to do with His property? The parable of the talents confirms that God expects you to use His prop-erty wisely.

↪ How does 2 Peter 2:2 relate to the fact that our bodies belong to God?

Dear Lord, give me the strength today to live in such a way that will honor You.

Father God, forgive me for the times I have allowed my lack of control to dishonor You in any way.

DAY 4: *The Price Tag on Your Life*

How do you know what something is worth? In a free-market system, value is determined by the price the highest bidder will pay for an item. How do we know what our lives are worth? We can simply ask, "What price was paid?" The startling answer is: "You are extremely valuable to God because He paid *the* extreme price for you!" (see 1 Corinthians 6:20).

Read the following Scripture passages and then write the words from the verses that show you that you are valuable.

Scripture	I know I am valuable because...
Romans 5:10	
Romans 8:32	
Galatians 1:4	
Galatians 2:20	
1 Timothy 2:6	
Titus 2:14	
Hebrews 7:27	
Hebrews 9:28	
1 John 2:2	

God paid a high price for you—you are extremely valuable. Now you are profoundly responsible for what you do with your life. Offer your life to God as a sacrifice.

➣ What does Hebrews 13:15,16 say about sacrifices that are pleasing to God?

≫ Write a prayer of praise to God.

Lord, thank You for the sacrifice You made to atone for my sin. Thank You for not leaving me in the depths of my sin.

Lord God, help me to offer my body as a pleasing sacrifice to You. Let me continually offer up my sacrifice of praise and service.

DAY 5: *Honoring and Worshiping God*

≫ What does Revelation 4:11 have to say about honoring God?

≫ According to 1 Corinthians 6:19, how are you to honor God?

≫ How did the Christians described in 2 Corinthians 8:23 do this?

By the way these Corinthian Christians lived, they not only represented their churches well, they also brought honor to Christ. People thought highly of Christ because of their actions. One of the ways to honor Christ is the way you control your body.

➺ What do you think is meant by "control his own body" in
1 Thessalonians 4:4?

Another reason your body is valuable is because you, through your
body, can worship God.

➺ What does Romans 12:1 say about your body and honoring God?

➺ Read Titus 3:4,5. Write a prayer thanking God that He has not given
you what you deserve, but instead He has given you mercy.

➺ As you meet your goals in the First Place program, how can those
accomplishments become something that honors Christ?

➺ According to Galatians 5:22,23, what is one evidence that Christ is
working in you?

 Lord, help me to honor you today through self-control.
God, help me daily to offer my body as a living sacrifice
that is holy and pleasing to You.

DAY 6: *Reflections*

In this week's Bible study, we focused on the value of our bodies as temples of the Holy Spirit. Your heart is the soul of the Spirit and your mind bears the evidence of the Holy Spirit as He guides your words and actions.

Both the heart and mind must be filled with the Spirit to effectively fight the battles against your enemy, Satan. What you put into your mind will manifest itself in your heart and actions. Fill your mind with those things that are pleasing to God. In that way, you will build a temple of both physical and spiritual beauty.

Although God wants you to be healthy, He is more concerned about the physical beauty that comes from loving Him, knowing His Word and obeying His commands. Through the First Place program you will energize your physical body, strengthen your mind, renew your Spirit and satisfy your emotional needs. Any weight loss you experience and any improvement in your physical body come as natural results and are extra blessings.

The way to that healthy body and mind that are pleasing to God is through knowing His Word. Memorizing and quoting Scripture such as this week's verse will give you added strength whenever you face temptation. With Scripture memory as part of your commitments in the First Place program, you will study and learn more about carrying out God's will for your life. Set a goal of learning one extra verse a week in addition to your memory verse. See how quickly your knowledge of Scripture builds.

The following are verses that Beth Moore used in *Praying God's Word* in the chapter on overcoming your enemy, Satan.

My faithful Father, help me to have absolute assurance that I am a child of God because the whole world system is presently under the control of the evil one (see 1 John 5:19).[1]

Father God, thank You for making me alive with Christ when I was dead in my sins and in the uncircumcision of my sinful nature. You forgave me all my sins, having canceled the written code, with its regulations, that was against me and that stood opposed to me. Christ took it away, nailing it to His cross. And having disarmed the powers and authorities,

Christ Jesus made a public spectacle of them, triumphing over them by the cross (see Colossians 2:13-15).[2]

I trust in You, Lord, so I'll let You rescue me. Teach me to delight in You and deliver me, O God (see Psalm 22:8).[3]

DAY 7: *Reflections*

When Solomon built the Temple, he made it a beautiful place filled with gold and precious materials. He wanted all the world to see its beauty and know that God filled it with His presence. When God created man and woman, He made the body a dwelling place for His Spirit for those who invite Him in. He wants all the world to see your beauty and know that His Holy Spirit lives in you.

Several of the verses studied this week referred to your body as a temple where the Spirit of God dwells. Since He chose you as a dwelling place, fill it with the good things that are pleasing and acceptable to Him. One of those pleasing and acceptable things is His Word. By filling your mind with the words of Scripture and writing them permanently on your heart, you are honoring God with your body.

The memory verse this week gives specific instruction about honoring God with your body. Jesus paid a great price to see that your sins would be forgiven, and you would have eternal life. In return God wants you to honor Him in all that you say and do.

As you complete this week's Bible study, repeat the memory verse. Each time you use the verse, God plants this Scripture more firmly in your mind and heart. You will be enabled to resist the temptations that come, knowing that God will provide the way out.

Lord Jesus, thank You for making me a temple and sending Your Spirit to live in me (see 1 Corinthians 3:16).

Only You are worthy, my Lord and God, to receive glory and honor and power, for You created all things, and by Your will they were created and have their being. Thank You for creating me in Your image (see Revelation 4:11).

Dear Heavenly Father, help me to remember that my body is a temple of the Holy Spirit who is in me, and whom I received from You. I am not my own because I was bought with a price. Therefore, I must honor You, O God, with my body (see 1 Corinthians 6:19,20).

Notes
1. Beth Moore, *Praying God's Word* (Nashville, TN: Broadman and Holman, 2000), p. 330.
2. Ibid., p. 329.
3. Ibid., p. 317.

GROUP PRAYER REQUESTS   TODAY'S DATE:_____

NAME	REQUEST	RESULTS

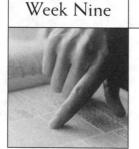

GOING GOD'S WAY

MEMORY VERSE
Commit to the LORD whatever you do,
and your plans will succeed.
Proverbs 16:3

A mother, frustrated by her child's disobedience, demanded that her seven-year-old son sit on a chair in the kitchen. Sensing he must obey or face unpleasant consequences, he sat. As he sat, the boy scowled and muttered to himself. After a few minutes, his mother asked, "What are you doing?" The boy replied, "I'm sitting on the outside, but I'm standing on the inside."

How do you respond to going God's way in life? Do you respond joyfully? Or do you resist God in stubborn rebellion?

In this week's study, you'll learn about the benefits of going God's way. You'll also discover harsh warnings about stiff-necked rebellion. You'll consider the advantages of following God's leadership in your life with a willing heart.

DAY 1: *Committing Your Way to God*

Could you pray, "God, I want what You want in my life" and truly mean it? The memory verse for the week tells you to commit to the Lord whatever you do, and you will succeed.

➤ To what degree could you or could you not honestly pray this prayer? What would keep you from praying this prayer?

We sometimes read a verse such as Proverbs 16:3 and say, "That's great. I'll decide what I want to do, commit those plans to the Lord, and God has promised to make me successful." Be careful. God hasn't promised to bless *your* plans. He promises to bless you when you walk in the path He has prepared for your life. Read Psalm 37:5,6 then answer the questions.

➤ What does it mean to "commit your way to the Lord"?

➤ How do you show trust in Him once you've committed your way to the Lord?

Once you commit your way to God, can you relax and trust Him? Or do you continue to worry about how the plans will unfold?

Choose the following statement that best describes you right now.

☐ I've learned to relax and trust God once I commit my way to Him.

☐ I end up somewhere in the middle: I commit my way, but I still worry.

☐ I can't seem to commit my way to Christ. I need to be in control.

➤ Explain why you checked the box you did.

When you decide to follow God's way willingly, wonderful things can happen. God can lead you easily. You can follow Him, trusting that He is leading you into situations that will be best for you.

 As you read the following verses, choose one from each pair and explain what the verse you chose means to you at this point in your spiritual life.

Joy in receiving God's direction: Psalm 16:11 or Psalm 119:35

Commitment to deal with sin that hinders God's direction: Psalm 119:133 or Psalm 139:24

Trust in Christ to protect and lead you: Psalm 61:2 or Psalm 143:10

Many Christians struggle to fully commit their way to the Lord. You may be one of them. Over time as you learn more about His plans for your life, you will find it easier to trust Him. As in all areas of the Christian life, this is an area where you have lots of room for spiritual growth.

Heavenly Father, help me to trust You completely with the direction of my life.

Father, give me the ability to commit my way to You and trust that Your way is best.

DAY 2: *Fully Committed*

What does God hope to find as He surveys the world? According to
2 Chronicles 16:9, He looks for fully committed followers.

≫ If God were surveying the world, making a list of people with hearts
fully committed to Him, would He add you to His list? Why or why
not?

≫ We know we are fully committed to giving Christ first place in our
lives by our readiness to obey God's commands. How willing are you
to obey Christ?

≫ On one occasion, King Solomon challenged the people of Israel with
the words found in 1 Kings 8:61. After reading the verse, describe
where you are right now in this area of commitment.

≫ Perhaps you are willing to obey but doubt you have the strength
to obey. Read the following verses and write the promise found
in each one:

The promise in Psalm 28:7 is

The promise in Jeremiah 33:3 is

The promise in Philippians 4:13 is

➺ How do you feel about your commitments to First Place after 9 or 10 weeks?

➺ How do you feel about reading the Bible? Does Psalm 1:2 describe your attitude?

➺ How do you feel about the time spent in Bible study with the Lord each day?

➺ What does Psalm 37:4 promise when you "delight yourself in the Lord"?

God promises that you can do everything through the strength He gives you. His strength becomes a shield that protects you. Decide today to follow the path God has set for you.

Heavenly Father, I thank You for the promises You give to strengthen me today as I commit my life to You.

Precious Lord and Savior, I thank You for giving me direction in my life and sing praises to You for the progress I am making in trusting You completely.

Day 3: A Willing Spirit

The Bible refers to King David as a man after God's own heart (see Acts 13:22). Yet David sinned against God, then compounded the problem through stubborn rebellion. But when God's prophet Nathan confronted David with his sin, David repented and returned once again to following God's way. He recorded his experience in Psalm 51. Psalm 51:12 expresses a key to David's spiritual renewal.

⇒ How would your life as a Christian change if God gave you a willing spirit?

⇒ How would a willing spirit help you do the things you need to do as part of the First Place program?

God works in our lives to discipline us when we stray from His path. When that discipline occurs, we need to respond appropriately. Your attitude towards God's discipline makes a big difference in how successful you will be at changing your lifestyle and being obedient to God. He wants only the best for you, but sometimes you may feel rebellious because you want to be in control. Relax, and let God lead you. His control is not meant to chain you to hard rules but to set you free to enjoy the life He has planned for you.

⇒ According to Hebrews 12:5,6, how should you respond when God disciplines you?

⇒ According to Hebrews 12:10,11, what can you expect God's discipline to accomplish in your life?

Once you decide to go God's way, you will find wonderful things will happen. God can lead you easily. You can follow Him, trusting that He is leading you into situations that will be best for you. God allowed Satan to destroy Job's health, his family, his wealth; but Job stood steadfast in the Lord. He never wavered from seeking and submitting himself to God.

➤ What does Job 22:21 say is the result of submission to God?

Always be on guard against your enemy, the devil. Satan delights in seeing you suffer and turn to your own ways. But God is faithfully standing beside you; and when the Lord is in control, Satan will find it a difficult, if not impossible, task to make you stumble. If you are like many Christians, you want God in control of your life, but your desires may be holding you back. Peter loved Jesus and followed Him willingly, but just as Jesus told Peter to watch and pray, so must you.

➤ In Matthew 26:41, what did Jesus tell Peter to do? How is this a warning to you?

Perhaps you are willing to do what you know you should do, but have a weak spirit. Don't be ashamed; even the most obedient believers stray at times. But God is with you, and He will set you back on the path and give you a willing spirit.

 Dear Lord, You know my heart, and I ask You today to help me submit to Your discipline willingly and without resistance.

Father God, shore me up and give me courage so that when my spirit is weak, I am willing submit to You.

DAY 4: A Rebellious Spirit

God warns strongly about the danger of a rebellious spirit. He deals harshly with those who resist His plans. You may not think of yourself as rebelling against God. You may say you have a strong personality, or you think you know what is right for you. In reality, you might be rebelling against God's plans.

A teenage girl wanted to be a missionary. Every time the invitation came for those called to the mission field, she went forward, but she didn't feel God's call. Still she went forward and volunteered for special service in any way God wanted to use her. Several years later, after graduating from college, she entered a career, but felt unfulfilled. She still wanted to be a missionary. She applied for admission to a seminary and was accepted. She quit her job and prepared for the move. However, she still didn't feel at peace with her decision. She finally broke down and prayed, "God, I want to do what you want me to do, but I don't know what it is. I quit my job to go to seminary. If that's not what You want, tell me. If I am offered another job here, then I will stay and wait for Your direction." She received a job offer that afternoon, stayed where she was and began teaching school and working with youth at her church. She found her mission field close to home.

➵ This girl was being rebellious by trying to do what she thought God wanted, rather than seek His true direction. Read the following verses and write the biblical truth about spiritual rebellion.

Scripture	Biblical Principle About Spiritual Rebellion
Deuteronomy 9:24	
Job 24:13	
Psalm 25:7	
Psalm 106:43	

Scripture	Biblical Principle About Spiritual Rebellion
Psalm 107:11	
Isaiah 30:9	
Ezekiel 12:2	
Hosea 14:9	

➤ Do you have a rebellious spirit? How does this spirit demonstrate itself in the First Place program?

Many areas in the First Place program give rise to rebellion. Unwillingness to exercise or to fill out the Commitment Record, not eating the right foods, waiting to do all the Bible study at one time and resistance to memorizing Scripture may all be forms of rebellion against a program that you may feel is telling you what to do rather than doing what you feel is right. Think about why you joined First Place and about your motives for participation. Trying to lose weight by yourself has probably failed, but you don't want to admit it.

➤ As you near the end of this 13-week session, how successful have you been in overcoming your rebellion? What has First Place meant to you?

Lord, forgive me for any rebellious spirit that keeps me from obeying Your commands and fully committing my way to You.

Lord God, I praise Your holy name because You don't give up on me. You continue to love me and guide me even when I stray from the plan you set before me.

DAY 5: *Stiff-Necked and Stubborn*

God used graphic word pictures in the Bible to help us understand rebelliousness. The images God used to describe rebellious hearts should make us evaluate our lives and make tough changes. Read the following verses and answer the questions.

» Isaiah 48:4: In what ways do you respond to God with stiff-necked resistance?

» Jeremiah 7:24: In what areas of your life are you going spiritually backward, rather than forward, due to stubbornness on your part?

» Hosea 4:16: Notice the contrast between the stubborn heifers and the lambs. What is this word picture telling you?

» Acts 7:51: How did Stephen describe the Jewish religious leaders who resisted the Holy Spirit?

If any of these verses describes you, don't be discouraged. Ask God to show you the way to remove the stubbornness. You must guard against resisting God's work in your life. As a Christian, God's Spirit is continually working in you. You must respond obediently to Him and commit your paths to Him.

≫ Identify any areas of your life right now in which you are resisting God's Holy Spirit and the changes He wants to make in your life.

≫ Read Psalm 119:47 aloud. Has it become easier for you to obey God's commands? Can you say the words of this verse and mean them? Why or why not?

Lord, give me an obedient spirit that delights itself in Your commands because I love You.

God, forgive me for the times I have been unwilling to make changes You have wanted me to make. I trust You for the strength to do what I should do.

DAY 6: *Reflections*

This week's study focused on going God's way and committing your life to Him. God desires for you to have a willing spirit as you commit your ways to Him. He will forgive the times when you were unwilling to make changes if you come to Him and ask His forgiveness for your rebellious heart.

In order to be fully committed to God's purpose in your life, you must read and search the Scriptures for instructions for living. You have completed nine weeks of studying the Bible and learning how to have victories in your life.

Prayer, Bible study and Scripture memorization are the keys to knowing what God wants to do in your life. Have you been memorizing Scripture? If not, then commit yourself now to going back and writing the words of your memory verses in your heart.

In your prayer time, use the verses from the Bible studies to help you seek God's guidance. Offer your prayers of supplication in the words of the Bible. They will be more powerful against Satan than you can ever imagine.

We have referred to Beth Moore's book *Praying God's Word* because it is an excellent resource to use in learning to overcome the strongholds that threaten to undermine your willingness to obey God. The following verses concern overcoming strongholds related to the First Place program.

God, according to Your liberating Word, I was called to be free. Help me not to use my freedom to indulge my sinful nature; rather, I should serve others in love (see Galatians 5:13).

Lord, I have too long given the devil a foothold. Please help me to stop offering him so many opportunities to bring defeat into my life. Your plan for me is victory (see Ephesians 4:27).

My faithful Father, whether I turn to the right or to the left, cause my ears to hear a voice behind me saying, "This is the way; walk in it" (see Isaiah 30:21).[1]

DAY 7: *Reflections*

Decide today to go God's way in life. Decide to delight in His laws and His ways. Decide today to do whatever God asks you to do, knowing it will be the best plan for you. Spend some time talking with God about your commitments to Him. Trust Him to seal the commitments you are making and to give you the strength to keep them.

Even though this 13-week session is almost over, you still have time to commit yourself to carrying out God's plan for your life. Continue with your Bible study, Scripture memory and prayer time. Listen to the CD and use the Scripture memory cards to reinforce what you have learned this session.

Each week, the seventh day of your Bible study has ended with a prayer written from the memory verse for that week. Review those prayers and use them in your own prayer time to strengthen your will to follow God's plan for you. You should be well on your way to overcoming any strongholds that threaten to keep you from following God's will for your life. Don't be discouraged if you slip, for God is your refuge and fortress. Go to Him with your disappointments, anger, resentment, guilt, depression or whatever might threaten you. He will forgive and help you overcome.

 Lord God, Your divine power has given me everything I need for life and godliness through my knowledge of You who called me by Your own glory and goodness (see 2 Peter 1:3).

You, O Lord, have filled my heart with greater joy than when my grain and new wine abound (see Psalm 4:7).

Lord, I commit to You everything I do because I know that You help me to succeed (see Proverbs 16:3).

Note
1. Beth Moore, *Praying God's Word* (Nashville, TN: Broadman and Holman, 2000), pp. 155, 156, 158.

GROUP PRAYER REQUESTS   TODAY'S DATE:_____

NAME	REQUEST	RESULTS

WITHOUT LOVE–NOTHING

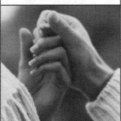

MEMORY VERSE

A new command I give you: Love one another.
As I have loved you, so you must love one another.
By this all men will know that you are my disciples,
if you love one another.
John 13:34,35

Historian Arnold Toynbee said, "I think that love is the only spiritual power that can overcome the self-centeredness that is inherent in being alive. Love is the thing that makes life possible or, indeed, tolerable."

For many, life is intolerable because they don't believe anyone loves them. Yet God proclaims His love for every one of us. God wants you to receive His love. God expects you to share His love with others.

Nothing you do in life means anything without love—that includes reaching your goals in the First Place program. This week you'll learn more about love: God's love for you and your love for others.

DAY 1: *Love Begins with God*

Charles Galloway describes the need for love this way:

> The need to love and be loved is the simplest of all human wants. Man needs love like he needs the sun and the rain. He perishes without it. His basic longing is to be the object of love and to be able to give love. No other need is quite so significant to his nature.

So what *is* love? Let's investigate!

Read 1 John 4:10 and rewrite it in your own words.

God defines love by His actions. Without God's active demonstration of love, we would never know what it means to love. Without God's revelation, we might think of love only as an emotion. In reality, emotion is only part of love. God taught that love is active; love takes initiative.

According to John 3:16, how did God demonstrate His love for you?

What is the extent of God's love? Who is included in the circle of His love?

You can hear of God's love for the world and for you yet fail to grasp the reality of that love. Even for Christians, God's love exceeds comprehension. Answer the following questions based on Ephesians 3:17-19.

How wide is God's love? Think about the extent of God's love. Who can be included in the expanse of God's love?

How long is God's love? Think of the duration of God's love. How long will God keep loving the world? Loving you?

➣ **How high is God's love?** Think of the highest expressions of God's love. Think of the cross of Christ. What does the Cross tell you of God's love?

➣ **How deep is God's love?** Think of the depths to which God's love can reach. Can people sink so low in sin that God's love will not stoop to reach them?

Think about it. The God of the universe loves you! He sacrificed His only Son to make atonement for your sins. Because of His great love, You have eternal life.

Father God, teach me more about Your love and allow me to live this day with the awareness of that love.

Heavenly Father, thank You for loving me enough to send Your Son to take my place on the Cross and for giving me eternal life.

DAY 2: *Valuable to God*

One of the early Christian theologians, Augustine, said, "God loves each of us as if there were only one of us." That sounds wonderful, but how can we know that we truly are important to God?

➣ Jesus used three word pictures to describe God's love for us. How does each of the following describe your value to God?

The lilies in Matthew 6:28-31

The sparrows in Matthew 10:29-31

The lost sheep in Luke 15:3-7

If this is how much God cares for the lilies of the field, how much more God loves you. If this is how much God cares for the sparrows, how much more God loves you. If this is how much a shepherd cares for a lost sheep, how much more God loves you.

However, because God loves us, He commands that we love one another.

⇛ In Matthew 5:43,44, what does Jesus say about loving others?

Christians must love one another in all situations. Think about people you know who are difficult to love. Read 1 Corinthians 13:4-7 for a familiar definition of what love is and does.

⇛ The key words in 1 Corinthians 13:4-7 are listed in the following chart. To the right of each word, write a practical application of how you can demonstrate love for some of the people in your life.

Practical Love for Difficult People		
Key Word	**How I Will Express Love**	
patient	I will be patient with	even when
kind	I will be kind to	even when
envy	I will not envy	even when

Practical Love for Difficult People		
Key Word	**How I Will Express Love**	
rude	I will not be rude with	even when
angry	I will not be angry with	even when
protect	I will protect especially	even when
trust	I will trust	especially when

You can know with certainty that you are valued and loved by God because God has demonstrated His love toward you. Because of His love for you, you are expected to love others. Think of the one person who presents the greatest challenge to you. Ask God to give you the opportunity to express love in a practical way to that person today.

Father God, because of what is written in the Bible, I believe You love me and value me, but sometimes I struggle to believe it's true. Help me to feel and know Your love for me.

Heavenly Father, help me to love those with whom I find it difficult to get along.

DAY 3: *Love That Can't Be Earned*

A commercial for a financial services firm made this statement: "We make money the old-fashioned way; we earn it." Unfortunately, many people think that this principle applies to God's love. They believe they must earn God's love. The Bible states, however, that we cannot earn God's love.

➣ What does Romans 5:6-8 mean to you?

➤ Since Christ died for you while you were still a sinner, you could not have earned His love. How does this make you feel?

Some Christians live with the fear that although Christ may have loved them in the past, He may stop loving them in the future.

➤ Do you think God could stop loving you? Why or why not?

➤ How would your attitude about yourself and your life change if you were convinced that God loves you and nothing will ever make Him stop loving you?

➤ Why should 1 John 4:9,10 convince you that God loves you?

➤ What does Romans 8:35-37 say about the love of God?

With all of these promises and assurances concerning God's love, you can be certain that you will always be loved by God. You are one of His children. You can do nothing to earn His love; it is a gift of God to you as an heir to His kingdom.

Father God, thank You for Your unconditional love for me, a love I could never earn or deserve.

Lord Jesus, I love You and know that I am secure in Your love, because I have believed in You as the one who died for my sins and took my place on the Cross.

DAY 4: *Sharing God's Love*

On Day Two you learned that because you have received unconditional love from God, He expects you to respond by loving others. Love is much easier to affirm than to live. Perhaps you occasionally feel like Linus in the Peanuts cartoon who said, "I love mankind—it's people I can't stand."

➤ According to 1 John 4:11, why must we love others?

Those who have experienced God's love must share that love with others. God didn't intend for you to hoard His love. Love, especially God's love, must be given away.

Read John 13:34,35 and answer the following questions.

➤ What is the standard you should use as you seek to love others?

➤ What will others know when they see your love?

➤ What evidence indicates that God's love is flowing through your life to others?

Sometimes God sends tough situations in which you find it difficult to express love. First Corinthians 13:4-7 provides a helpful blueprint for you. With this list, you can focus on actions you should take in difficult situations. Once you know what you should do, you can trust God to give you strength to do the right thing.

Practical Love in Tough Situations	
Key Word	**How I Will Express Love**
boast	I will not boast about _____ even when
pride	I will not be prideful even if
self-seeking	I will not be self-seeking when
wrongs	I will not keep a record of wrongs, even about
evil	I will not delight when bad things happen to
truth	I will rejoice when the truth comes out even if
hope	I will not lose hope even if
persevere	I will persevere even if

God will help you demonstrate His love in the situations you will face in your life today. Trust Him to give you love so you can allow His love to flow through you.

God, I pray that Your love will flow through me and transform all that I do today.

Heavenly Father, allow me to experience Your love in such a way that I can share it with those who come into my life today.

DAY 5: *Anything Minus Love Equals Nothing*

Love is practical, active. One writer described love this way:

What does love look like? It has hands to help others. It has feet to hasten to the poor and needy. It has eyes to see misery and want. It has ears to hear my sighs and sorrows. That is what love looks like.

Love meets needs. But love is more than action. Actions without love are useless. Colossians 3:12-14 describes actions filled with love.

➤ What is one of the purposes of love described in verse 14?

Without love, the virtues of compassion, kindness, humility, gentleness, patience and forgiveness become hollow and fruitless. Love brings the perfect unity that only God can give.

➤ List the good actions described in 1 Corinthians 13:1-3.

This is an impressive list of activities. Yet without love, these activities count for nothing. Here's an equation: Anything minus love equals nothing. This love equation even extends to positive activities such as the First Place program.

Think about your goals in the First Place program. Consider what you are doing in light of the love equation and check the appropriate box after each statement:

≫ Have you treated your family in a loving way while you have been working to reach your First Place goals?   Yes ☐   No ☐

≫ Have you treated people where you work, at church or in other places in a loving way while you have been working through this program?   Yes ☐   No ☐

If you checked no to either question, God can help you change your behavior. He will help you to respond in love to the people in your life no matter what goals you are pursuing or what changes you are undergoing.

Heavenly Father, if I do anything without love, then it counts as nothing. Help me to show love to others in everything I do and say.

Lord, give me the opportunity today to show love through my actions.

DAY 6: *Reflections*

You have reached the last two days of study for this session. Throughout the study the emphasis has been on giving Christ first place in your heart, mind and life. Without Him you are nothing, but with Him in your life, you are a valued child of God.

You have learned how to pray, how to joyfully obey, how to please God, how to seek true satisfaction, how to get help in time of temptation and how to value your body and take care of it. Each week a memory verse has pointed you towards giving Christ first place in your life.

Now comes the time when you must truly put the principles found in these lessons to the test. They must become an integral part of your life.

Prayer, Bible study, Scripture reading and healthy eating and living habits need to continue to grow as you seek intimate relationship with God.

Look up the verses you have written in your prayer journal. If you haven't started a prayer journal or you haven't written down special verses, you can begin now. Recall times when a specific passage of Scripture helped you discover God's will for a particular situation, pulled you through a difficult time or helped you resist temptation. These verses that have special meaning for you are a good place to start when memorizing specific Scriptures. Add the following verses to your collection of memorized verses.

Lord God, You have shown me that even if I give all I possess to the poor and surrender my own body to the flames, but have not love, I am nothing, and I gain nothing (see 1 Corinthians 13:3).

Holy Lord, I am convinced that neither death nor life, neither angels, nor demons, neither the present nor the future, nor any powers, neither height, nor depth, nor anything else in all creation, will be able to separate me from the love of God that comes through Christ Jesus my Lord (see Romans 8:38,39).

DAY 7: *Reflections*

As this session of your First Place program ends, reflect on the many things you have learned about yourself and God. He is a God of love who wants the very best for all of His children. This past week you have read Scripture that affirms the mighty love He has for you and how He wants you to share that love with others. We wish you continued success as you live in step with what you have learned these past several weeks. Our prayers go with you.

The commitments of First Place are not just things you do while you're in this program. They should become a part of your daily life whether you're enrolled in a session or not. A life filled with Bible study, Scripture memorization, prayer, healthy eating, exercise and encouragement to others will keep you close to Him and feeling better about yourself.

If any stronghold still threatens to undermine your efforts to continue in the First Place program, review your memory verses and other Scripture used in this session. Use the verses as you pray for God to take control of your desires and lead you. By so doing, you will truly give Christ *first place* in your life.

Select two or three of your own special verses and write a prayer based on each one.

1.

2.

3.

 Holy God, help me to love others as You have loved me. Let all men know I am Your disciple through my love for others (see John 13:34,35).

Group Prayer Requests   Today's Date:_____

Name	Request	Results

BEING A GOOD GROUP MEMBER

One of the great things about First Place is *you don't have to go it alone!* It's not always easy making changes in your lifestyle, but with the support of others you are more likely to be successful in reaching your goals for healthy weight, good nutrition and effective living. In fact, studies indicate that long-term maintenance of weight loss and a healthy lifestyle are enhanced by commitment to and participation in a supportive group. There is definitely strength in numbers (see Ecclesiastes 4:9-12).

Much of the success of First Place comes because of the fellowship, prayers and support of your group. Your First Place group is a great source of encouragement and inspiration. Likewise, you will provide encouragement, inspiration, motivation and ideas to others. *Never underestimate the power of your prayers and support for the members of your group—and the support and prayers of others for you.* The success of your group depends on a cooperative team spirit and your active participation. Being a good group member gives you the opportunity to practice loving your neighbor as yourself (see Matthew 22:39).

Participating in a First Place group is an important responsibility. Many people are dealing with issues that run much deeper than weight loss alone. In addition to the nine First Place commitments, prayerfully commit to accepting help from members of your group and giving help to the members of your group.

THE BENEFITS OF PARTICIPATING IN YOUR FIRST PLACE GROUP

Your group is your support team. Discussing your feelings and experiences and listening to others help everyone to realize that none of us are alone. In a successful group, everyone feels safe and comfortable in expressing his or her thoughts and feelings. It's a group where everyone is able to freely share experiences, ask questions and offer solutions to problems.

First Place provides you with a good source of accountability and a supportive environment of fellow Christians who share in and understand your struggles and needs. Your group will help you keep things in perspective—emotionally, spiritually and physically.

Allowing Others to Help You

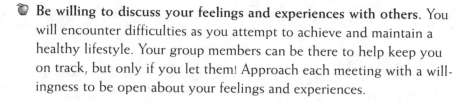

- **Be willing to discuss your feelings and experiences with others.** You will encounter difficulties as you attempt to achieve and maintain a healthy lifestyle. Your group members can be there to help keep you on track, but only if you let them! Approach each meeting with a willingness to be open about your feelings and experiences.

- **Never miss a meeting because you feel like you've blown it.** This is when your group will help you the most. One of the keys to successful weight loss is recognizing that you need the support of others—and then being open to letting them help.

- **Try to be optimistic and positive as often as you can.** Feel good about yourself and others in your group. Be open and honest, but look for the positives when you can. Be open to and appreciative of the support, encouragement, ideas and advice of others.

- **Try to develop a more personal relationship with one or more members of your group.** This person should be someone you are comfortable sharing with on a deeper level. However, do not allow this relationship to interfere with your participation in the group.

- **Participate at a level that's comfortable for you.** Not everyone is completely comfortable in a group setting—that's okay. Before attending each meeting, prayerfully consider ways you can open up and participate. Let your group leader and your group know how you are feeling.

Helping Others in Your Group

- **Regular attendance demonstrates your commitment to the group.** When you miss a meeting, other members worry about you. When you miss regularly, they may begin to think you don't care. Sometimes missing a meeting or being late is inevitable, but try to let your group leader or another member know when you are going to miss or be late.

- **Always try to arrive on time.** Arriving late disrupts the flow of the meeting and causes you to miss important information. If you notice someone else missing frequently or always running late, ask if you can help.

- **Give the group your full attention.** Listen to what others have to say. Look at others while they're speaking. Try not to interrupt when others are talking. Try to identify what they're expressing and feeling. Offer suggestions and support when you can.

- **Never judge or respond to other members in a negative way.** Your job is to offer prayers, support and helpful advice. What another member is experiencing or feeling is important, even if you don't understand or agree. Help create an environment in which others are comfortable sharing their feelings and experiences. Be happy for the success of others.

- **Monitor your feelings and reactions to other members of your group.** Naturally, there will be some members you like and understand more than others, but don't allow negative feelings influence how you treat another member. Try to identify the source of your feelings and prayerfully consider ways to overcome your feelings.

- **Always keep personal information of others confidential.** Always get another member's permission before you share any personal information with anyone else.

Asian restaurants have become an American favorite. With a variety of foods, cooking styles and atmospheres, they offer both enjoyable and healthful dining. Asian restaurants often use low-fat cooking methods and lean meats, fresh vegetables, rice and noodles. However, these same nutritious foods are often deep fried or stir fried and served with high-sodium sauces. Add in the typically large portions and an egg roll and a single meal can easily top 1500 calories.

WHAT SHOULD I ORDER?

With the diversity of Asian cuisine—Chinese, Japanese, Thai and Vietnamese—and cooking styles, it's important to know how to read menus. The following chart of the most common menu items and terms will aid you in choosing wisely. Choose low-fat items more often and high-fat and high-sodium items less often.

Low in fat	High in Fat	High in Sodium
Water chestnuts	Tempura	Black bean sauce
Simmered	Duck	Hoisin sauce
Barbecued	Wonton	Miso sauce
Bean curd	Peanuts or cashews	Most soups
Steamed	Fried rice or noodles	Oyster sauce
Braised	Coconut milk	Pickled
Roasted or grilled	Fried or crispy	Soy sauce
Stir fried	Egg rolls	Teriyaki sauce

Did You Know?

🍎 Some Asian sauces, such as sweet-and-sour and plum sauce, are actually low in fat, calories and sodium. The problem is that dishes served with these sauces often consist of deep fried meats.

A tablespoon of soy sauce has nearly 1,000 milligrams of sodium—almost half of the recommended daily intake of 2,400 milligrams.

 While Asian cuisine uses lots of vegetables, salads are somewhat unusual. The exceptions are Thai and Vietnamese cuisine which offer a variety of salads, including garden salads.

 The trendy Japanese sushi—a combination of raw fish, vinegared rice and often seaweed—is actually low in fat, calories and sodium, depending on the dipping sauce.

HEALTHY CHOICES FOR ANY OCCASION

Appetizers and Soups

 Traditional appetizers such as egg rolls, wonton and fried shrimp are high in calories and fat. Ask if the restaurant offers steamed spring rolls or steamed dumplings instead. If you choose the egg roll, eat only the filling.

 Many Asian soups, such as hot-and-sour and egg-drop, offer a great way to start a meal. These broth-based soups are low in calories and fat.

The Main Meal

Asian dishes are usually served in large portions—enough for at least two people. Remember a serving of rice is one-third of a cup! Ask for a to-go box before your meal and store away the extra portions for another meal. It's usually a good idea to order fewer dishes than people and then share them family style.

Choose the following dishes:
- Dishes with steamed rice or noodles
- Steamed fish, stir-fried chicken or other lean meats
- Stir-fried dishes with fresh vegetables such as broccoli, cabbage, carrots, water chestnuts, mushrooms and sprouts. Try tofu!
- For dessert, have the fortune cookie if you want. Coconut desserts can be high in fat and calories.

Choose the following dishes less often:

- Fried rice, noodles, egg rolls and wonton

- Breaded and fried meats found in tempura or sweet-and-sour sauce. Ask how the meat is prepared before ordering.

- Dishes with cashews or peanuts—ask that the amount of nuts be cut in half.

Other Tips to Remember

🍎 Let family or friends who are dining with you know that you plan to eat healthy. Order what you know is best for you and don't let others tempt you into ordering less healthy foods.

🍎 Become familiar with a few restaurants you enjoy where you know you can order healthy foods. Learn to make special requests like substituting steamed rice for fried rice. Ask that your meal be prepared with less oil or fewer added fats. Avoid restaurants or foods that can tempt you from your plan.

🍎 If you order an item that is higher in fat, balance it with a low-fat choice, such as steamed rice or steamed vegetables.

🍎 Ask that stir-fry and other dishes be cooked with very little oil.

🍎 Be careful when eating Asian food buffet style. Plan to make healthy choices and select reasonable portions.

🍎 When eating take-out food at home, serve what you need on a plate and store the rest.

GETTING STARTED

List the Asian restaurants where you dine most often. Next, list the foods that you usually order. Now, what can you change to make your meals healthier? Use the table on the following page to help you plan for healthy choices the next time you eat Asian food.

Restaurant	Usual Choices (Be specific)	Better Choices (Be specific)

JOIN THE CLUB

TIPS FOR SELECTING A FITNESS CENTER

Are you looking for the best way to fit physical activity into your life? There is no *one* best way. The best way is the one that works for you. Joining a fitness center can be a great choice for some people. Fitness centers offer a wide selection of equipment and activities to help you achieve and maintain a physically active lifestyle and all the benefits that go along with it. They also provide a safe and comfortable environment in all kinds of weather, almost any time of the day.

IS JOINING A FITNESS CENTER RIGHT FOR ME?

You have several options when it comes to fitting physical activity into your life. You can purchase home exercise equipment, exercise outdoors, walk in the mall or fit *lifestyle* physical activities into your daily routine (i.e., taking the stairs instead of the elevator, working in your yard, etc.). The most important thing is to choose activities that you enjoy and that fit into your lifestyle. Before joining a fitness center, ask yourself the following questions:

	Yes	No
Have I been a member of a fitness center before?		
If yes, did I enjoy and use it regularly?		
Can I afford all the fees (initiation, membership and classes)?		
Is there a fitness center close to my home or work?		
Do I have the time to use a fitness center regularly?		
Do I enjoy working out with others?		
Do I enjoy having a wide variety of exercise options from which to choose?		
Will I benefit from having an expert staff of fitness professionals to help me choose and maintain an effective, safe physical activity program?		
Will joining a fitness center provide the motivation and inspiration I need to get and stay active?		
What specific benefits (i.e., equipment, group classes, supervision or amenities) am I looking for from a fitness center? List them:		

How Do I Choose a Fitness Center That's Right for Me?

When selecting a fitness center, there are several important things to consider:

🍎 **Is it convenient?** Studies show that you are more likely to use a center if it's within 10 to 12 minutes of your home or workplace. Remember, lack of time and inconvenient location are two common reasons people give for dropping out of a fitness program!

🍎 **Does it provide a safe, friendly and comfortable environment?** Ask the club to allow you to work out for several days before joining— many clubs will. This helps you to see if you are comfortable in the club and enables you to become familiar with the equipment, staff and other members. If a club won't allow you a trial period, look elsewhere!

🍎 **Is the staff trained and certified in exercise instruction and counseling?** Among the top certifications are the American College of Sports Medicine, the American Counsel on Exercise and the National Strength and Conditioning Association.

🍎 **Do they offer classes for all levels of fitness and skill?** Make sure the club has classes at your level at convenient times for you.

🍎 **Does the center have a wide selection of exercise equipment?** Is the equipment clean and in good working order? Check for "out of order" signs. Check the size of the crowd at the time you will be using the facility, for availability of the equipment you'll want to use.

🍎 **What extra features are you looking for?** Do you want a swimming pool, racquet courts, locker rooms, private showers, massage services, steam rooms, hot tubs or cafeteria?

🍎 **How much are you willing to spend on a membership?** Do you want to pay monthly or annually?

🍎 **What special programs and services does the club offer**: child care, educational programs, nutritional counseling, personal training, etc.? Are these important to you?

THINGS TO LOOK OUT FOR

- **High-pressure sales techniques**: You need to have time to think about your decision and review the contract and terms of membership. If you feel pressured, that club's probably not for you!

- **Long-term contracts—longer than one year**: In fact, you may prefer a monthly membership at first to see if the fitness center is right for you.

- **Membership options and contracts that are hard to understand**

- **Fitness centers that don't ask you about your health and medical history**

- **Centers that appear to be understaffed**

TIPS FOR GETTING THE MOST OUT OF A FITNESS CENTER

- Ask the staff to give you an orientation to the center and the equipment. Staff should always be available to answer your questions and help you use the equipment safely and effectively.

- Choose a work-out time that's convenient for you. Schedule your exercise time just as you would any other important appointment.

- Choose activities and equipment you enjoy.

- Set specific goals for health and physical activity to keep you motivated.

- Get a loved one, coworker or friend to join you. The support of a buddy often keeps you on track.

- You may need to ask for help around the house or at work so you can fit in your workout.

NUTRITION
WHILE TRAVELING

Whether traveling for business or pleasure, eating healthy on the road can be difficult. The secret is *getting away* without *getting back* all the weight you've worked so hard *getting off.* With a little planning, you can keep on track when you travel.

How to Eat Healthy When Traveling

Part of the enjoyment of traveling is the chance to try out new cuisine. When you travel, allow yourself to enjoy new foods. A *few* choices that are higher in fat, sugar and calories are okay.

The key is to plan ahead how you want to eat while traveling and stick to it. Get support from your traveling companions. Let them know that you plan to eat healthy. It's much easier to make healthy choices when you have the support of others. Plus, you might be a positive influence on them!

Eating on the Road

- **Pack your own snacks.** Good choices include bagels, fresh or dried fruits, raw vegetables, low-fat crackers, rice cakes, pretzels and cereal bars. By having your own snacks with you, you can avoid becoming too hungry and then overeating the first chance you get.

- **Eat a healthy meal before you hit the road.** Filling up before you leave will help you avoid making less healthful choices while on the road.

- **Pack a cooler** full of sandwiches, fruits, vegetables, low-fat yogurt and healthy beverages such as water, juice and low-fat milk.

- **When eating at fast-food restaurants, avoid fried foods and supersize or deluxe meals.** Choose regular-size portions and choose grilled-chicken or other lean-meat sandwiches, baked potatoes (but easy on the cheese!) and fresh salads.

- **Stop regularly for a little physical activity,** such as stretching and a short walk—every little bit helps!

Eating in the Air

- **Don't eat the airline meal just because it's offered.** Ask yourself if you're hungry. What are your meal plans when you arrive? If you're not hungry or you're planning to eat when you arrive, save the calories. Instead, ask for milk or juice and a snack to curb your appetite.

- **Call at least 48 hours in advance to request a special meal:** low-fat, low-cholesterol or vegetarian.

- **Water is a great way to stay hydrated in the pressurized environment.** Choose fruit or vegetable juice, low-fat milk or water instead of soft drinks or other beverages. Water is a great way to stay hydrated while you're in the air.

- **Bring your own food in a carry-on bag.** Good choices include fresh and dried fruit, ready-to-eat cereals, bagels, crackers and low-fat cheese.

- **Eat a healthy meal or snack before you arrive at the airport or board the airplane.**

- **Walk around the airport,** not only to get a little exercise but also to stake out healthy food options.

- **When the "fasten seat belt" sign goes off, get up and walk** up and down the aisle every 20 minutes or so.

Eating Out on the Town

- **Choose restaurants wisely.** You can call the restaurant ahead of time to check out the menu. Ask if they prepare food to order or accept special requests.

- **Watch out for those large portions.** Try to choose smaller portions or share larger portions with a companion. Three ounces of meat is about the size of a deck of playing cards.

- **Don't skip meals to save up for that special meal.** Balance out a meal higher in fat and calories by making healthier choices during the day.

- **If you eat dessert, share it with a companion or take only a few bites.**

- **Beware of buffets.** Load up on fresh fruits, vegetables and other low-fat choices. Don't load up your plate just because it's "all you can eat." Rather than trying all the foods, pick one or two of your favorites and keep your portions small.

- **Eating smaller portions is a good way to enjoy a variety of foods.** Balance less healthy choices with better choices such as fresh fruits, vegetables and whole-grain foods.

- **When dining in foreign countries, you may need to avoid raw fruits and vegetables, raw or partly cooked meats and tap water.** A good rule to remember: If it's been boiled, cooked, bottled or peeled, it's probably okay.

Other Tips

- **Stay at hotels and resorts that offer healthy dining options.**

- **Start each day with a healthy breakfast.** Fresh fruit; toast, a bagel or English muffin with jam; hot or cold cereal; and low-fat yogurt are good choices. Fresh-squeezed juice and low-fat or nonfat milk are good beverage choices. Limit your intake of eggs, sausage, bacon, sweet rolls, donuts, croissants and fried potatoes.

- **Carry snacks with you to business meetings or while sight-seeing.** Try to avoid becoming overly hungry. If you wait too long between meals, you're more likely to overeat or make less healthy choices.

- **Make time for physical activity.**

➤ List a few healthy eating ideas you're ready to try on your next trip.

Hidden Fats

When eating away from home, it can be difficult to estimate how much fat is in a meal. It's important to estimate hidden fats in food because extra calories can add up quickly. Just one teaspoon of oil or one tablespoon of salad dressing has 5 grams of fat and 45 calories. Considering that a ladle of dressing at most salad bars is three or four tablespoons, it's easy to see how fat calories can add up!

- Vegetables cooked with oil or butter—add one-half to one fat exchange
- Any fried food (meat, vegetable, French fries)—add one to two fat exchanges
- Tuna, chicken or potato salad—add two fat exchanges
- Salad with regular dressing—add two fat exchanges
- Gravy and special sauces—add one fat exchange

The best way to control hidden fats when eating out is to ask that foods be prepared without added fats and that salad dressing, gravies and sauces be served on the side.

What steps are *you* ready to take to get control of the portion sizes you eat?

THE AMAZING 10-MINUTE WORKOUT

No time, no fun and *bo-or-or-ring!* These are common reasons people give for not making physical activity a lifetime habit. Yet experts are making it harder and harder to come up with good excuses. The latest recommendations tell us that exercise doesn't have to be hard to be beneficial. In fact, exercise doesn't even have to be exercise! Gone are the days when you had to exercise for at least 30 minutes at a certain heart rate to get the health and fitness benefits of aerobic exercise. What's the exercise prescription for today? "Something is better than nothing, and more is better than something."

The latest recommendations from groups such as the American Heart Association and the American College of Sports Medicine call for at least 30 minutes of moderate physical activity on as many days of the week as possible—preferably every day. The latest twist on this new recommendation is that the activity doesn't have to be done all at one time. Shorter amounts accumulated over the course of a day appear to offer the same health benefits as the more traditional 30 continuous minutes of exercise.

THE BENEFITS OF SHORTER WORKOUTS

Shorter workouts are easier to start and to stick with. It's easy to get burned out on exercise by doing too much too soon. Start slow and work your way up to longer sessions as your physical activity becomes a habit.

You may also be a person who just doesn't have 30 to 60 minutes to give at one time. Shorter workouts are easier to fit into your schedule and fight boredom by allowing more variety in your routine. They're also great for regular exercisers who occasionally miss or are unable to do their usual routine. When you miss or know you are going to miss a session, just slip in one or two of these shorter workouts wherever and whenever you can.

Are lack of time, lack of enjoyment and boredom among the reasons you have a hard time making exercise a part of your life? Whether you're a regular exerciser or just getting started, think about it. Consider some of the following ideas for fitting 10-minute workouts into your day:

- Walking can be done anywhere, anytime. Think about times in your typical day when you can fit in a short, brisk walk.

- Get up 10 minutes earlier and fit in a quick walk before starting your day.

- Walk as part of your daily quiet time.

- Take 10-minute walking breaks at work.

- Arrive to work 10 minutes early and walk or climb the stairs.

- Take a 10-minute walk around the mall before stopping to shop.

- Walk your dog for 10 minutes.

- Take the entire family out for a 10-minute walk before or after meals.

- Walk around the house during commercials or between shows—you'll easily get in 10 minutes.

Walking is not your only choice. Here are some other creative ideas:

- Pick up the pace when you're doing household chores: 10 minutes of vacuuming, washing the car or working in the yard add up over the course of a day. To get the benefit, however, you have to push the pace a bit. Turn on your favorite music to help keep you moving.

- Buy an exercise videotape and pop it in for 10 minutes.

- Do you have exercise equipment that's collecting dust? Pull it out and try a 10-minute routine instead of feeling like you have to stay on for 30 minutes or longer.

- Rather than just watching your kids play, spend 10 minutes playing with them: shoot baskets, throw a ball or Frisbee, kick a soccer ball, etc.

- Take 10-minute breaks at work and do calisthenics, strength training or stretching exercises.

➤ List a few activities that you enjoy and can do for approximately 10 minutes at a time. Be creative—don't limit yourself to the traditional exercises. Whatever you choose to do, try to make it fun. Remember, the E in exercise is for enjoyment!

➤ Now that you've chosen a few activities, think of some times you can fit them into your day. Think about times in your day when you can be more active, such as when you watch television, shop, work around the house or take a break.

Morning

Noon

Evening

➤ Who can help you free up 10 minutes of time in your daily schedule?

UNDERSTANDING PORTION CONTROL

Portion control may be one of the biggest factors causing the rising rate of obesity in this country. When it comes to food these days, bigger is better! There are "Super Meal Deals," "Supersize" and "50% more," and in many restaurants one meal is sometimes big enough to feed a family. Even too much of the right foods can make you gain weight. Learning appropriate portion sizes for different foods may be one of the most important skills you can learn when it comes to achieving and maintaining your healthy weight. It's a skill that takes time and practice to develop.

WHAT CAN YOU DO TO MASTER PORTION CONTROL?

- **Use the right tools.** Make sure you use measuring cups and spoons and a food scale to help you learn about the portion sizes you eat. These tools allow you to compare what you *really* eat with what you *should* eat. Measure all the foods you eat to learn about common servings.

- **Try eating with smaller plates and bowls.** This will help you avoid serving portions that are too large. It also makes smaller portions look bigger.

- **Cut foods, such as meat, into smaller pieces.** This also gives the appearance of more food and can help the meal last longer.

- **Buy meats and cheese that are already cut in appropriate serving sizes.**

- **Get out of the habit of eating everything on your plate, especially at restaurants.** Learn to stop eating before you're full; it's okay to leave some food behind. It's also okay to split a meal with a companion.

CONTROLLING MEAT, POULTRY AND FISH PORTIONS

One of the areas in which calories can easily add up unnoticed is the meat group. The recommended serving size for meat is three ounces.

Unfortunately, we've gotten used to eating two to three times this amount. This is especially challenging when eating in restaurants. The average portion of meat served when dining out is 6 to 10 ounces. Remember, too, that restaurants don't always offer the leanest cuts of meat. With all of this in mind, it is a good idea to learn how to estimate a 3-ounce portion of meat:

🍎 **Dinner-plate rule**: Imagine a standard dinner plate divided in quarters. Your meat serving should only fill one quarter of your plate. This means the other three-quarters should consist of complex carbohydrates—one-fourth starch and one-half vegetables/fruit.

3 OUNCES OF MEAT, POULTRY OR FISH = 1/4 OF THE PLATE

CARBOHYDRATES = 3/4 OF THE PLATE

🍎 **Deck of cards**: An old favorite when trying to estimate 3-ounce portions of meat. A 3-ounce portion of meat should be no thicker and no wider than a standard deck of cards.

🍎 **Lady's palm**: Three ounces of meat should fit nicely in the palm of an average-sized lady's palm.

🍎 **Eyeball rule**: This is another common rule. This is a simple rule of thumb that is easy to apply—if it looks too big, it probably is!

When grocery shopping, keep in mind that chicken breasts are typically closer to 5 or 6 ounces each. Individual filet mignons, although they look small, are at least 6- to 8-ounce portions. It's a good idea to plan on cutting these portions in half before preparing. Eating a couple of ounces more than you should can add at least 100 calories!

SHORTCUTS FOR ESTIMATING PORTION SIZES

The key to moderation is controlling portion size. To achieve and maintain healthy body weight, learn to put into practice the concepts of "serving size." Use measuring cups, spoons and scales until you know appropriate portion sizes by heart. Here are some practical examples from the American Dietetics Association to help you estimate portion sizes when these tools aren't available:

- A medium potato should be the size of a computer mouse.
- An average bagel should be the size of a hockey puck.
- A cup of fruit is the size of a baseball.
- A cup of lettuce is four leaves.
- Three ounces of meat is the size of an audiocassette.
- Three ounces of grilled fish is the size of a checkbook.
- One ounce of cheese is the size of four dice.
- One ounce of snack foods, such as pretzels, is one handful.

FIRST PLACE MENU PLANS

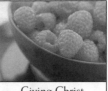

TWO WEEKS OF MENU PLANS

Each plan is based on approximately 1400 calories.

Breakfast	2 breads, 1 fruit, 1 milk, 0-½ fat (When a meat exchange is used, milk is omitted.)
Lunch	2 meats, 2 breads, 1 vegetable, 1 fruit, 1 fat
Dinner	3 meats, 2 breads, 2 vegetables, 1 fat
Snacks	1 bread, 1 fruit, 1 milk, ½-1 fat (or any remaining exchanges)

For more calories, add the following to the 1400 calorie plan.

1600 calories	Add 2 breads, 1 fat
1800 calories	2 meats, 3 breads, 1 vegetable, 1 fat
2000 calories	2 meats, 4 breads, 1 vegetable, 3 fats
2200 calories	2 meats, 5 breads, 1 vegetable, 1 fruit, 5 fats
2400 calories	2 meats, 6 breads, 2 vegetables, 1 fruit, 6 fats

The exchanges for these meals were calculated using the MasterCook software. It uses a database of over 6,000 food items prepared using United States Department of Agriculture (USDA) publications and information from food manufacturers. As with any nutritional program, MasterCook calculates the nutritional values of the recipes based on ingredients. Nutrition may vary due to how the food is prepared, where the food comes from, i.e., geography, soil content, season, ripeness, processing and method of preparation. For these reasons, please use the recipes and menu plans as approximate guides. As always consult your physician and/or a registered dietician before starting a diet program.

🍎 Breakfasts

2 reduced-fat frozen waffles
2 tsp. reduced-calorie maple syrup
1 tsp. low-calorie margarine
1 cup honeydew melon
1 cup nonfat milk

Exchanges: 2 breads, 1 fruit, 1 milk, ½ fat

~~~~~~

1 slice cinnamon-raisin toast
1 tsp. reduced-calorie margarine (to spread on toast)
½ tsp. granulated sugar and pinch of cinnamon (to sprinkle on toast)
¾ cup nonfat plain vanilla yogurt
¾ cup blueberries (to mix with yogurt)

Exchanges: 2 breads, 1 fruit, 1 milk, ½ fat

~~~~~~

1 small (2 oz.) whole-wheat English muffin, split and toasted
1 tsp. reduced-calorie margarine
1 cup strawberries, sliced
1 cup nonfat milk

Exchanges: 2 breads, 1 fruit, 1 milk, ½ fat

~~~~~~

2 slices reduced-calorie whole-wheat bread, toasted
1 tsp. reduced-calorie margarine
¾ cup corn flakes
½ medium banana, sliced
1 cup nonfat milk

Exchanges: 2 breads, 1 fruit, 1 milk, ½ fat

~~~~~~

2 slices reduced-calorie sourdough bread, toasted
1 tsp. reduced-calorie margarine
¾ cup blueberries
1 cup nonfat milk

Exchanges: 2 breads, 1 fruit, 1 milk, ½ fat

~~~~~~

1 cup fortified cold cereal

½ small mango

1 cup nonfat milk

Exchanges: 2 breads, 1 fruit, 1 milk

~~~~~~

1 small (2 oz.) bagel

1 tsp. strawberry jam

¾ cup artificially sweetened mixed-berry nonfat yogurt,

¾ cup blackberries (to mix in yogurt)

Exchanges: 2 breads, 1 fruit, 1 milk

~~~~~~

1 cup puffed rice cereal

½ medium banana, sliced

1 cup nonfat milk

Exchanges: 1 bread, 1 fruit, 1 milk

~~~~~~

1 small (2 oz.) English muffin

1 tsp. reduced-calorie margarine

½ medium grapefruit

1 cup nonfat milk

Exchanges: 2 breads, 1 fruit, 1 milk, ½ fat

~~~~~~

1 cup wheat flakes cereal

1 medium peach, sliced

1 cup nonfat milk

Exchanges: 2 breads, 1 fruit, 1 milk

~~~~~~

1 small (2 oz.) bagel, toasted

1 tsp. reduced-calorie margarine

¾ cup raspberries

1 cup nonfat milk

Exchanges: 2 breads, 1 fruit, 1 milk, ½ fat

~~~~~~

¾ cup bran flakes cereal

2 tbsp. raisins

1 cup nonfat milk

Exchanges: 2 breads, 1 fruit, 1 milk

~~~~~~

2 frozen pancakes, heated

2 tsp. low-calorie maple syrup

½ medium grapefruit

1 cup nonfat milk

Exchanges: 2 breads, 1 fruit, 1 milk, ½ fat

~~~~~~

¾ cup raisin-bran cereal

1 slice reduced-calorie wheat bread, toasted

1 tsp. reduced-calorie margarine

1 cup strawberries, sliced

1 cup nonfat milk

Exchanges: 2 breads, 1 fruit, 1 milk, ½ fat

~~~~~~

🍎 LUNCHES

Veggie Cheese Quesadillas

Nonstick cooking spray

2 6-inch nonfat flour tortillas

2 oz. reduced-fat Colby jack cheese, grated

1 tbsp. reduced-fat sour cream

½ cup frozen broccoli florets, cooked

¼ cup mushrooms, sliced

¼ cup salsa

Coat a nonstick skillet with cooking spray and heat. Put one tortilla in pan and sprinkle with cheese. Place broccoli and mushrooms on top of cheese. Cover with the second tortilla and brown on both sides. Remove from the pan and let sit a minute. Slice and serve with sour cream and salsa.

Serve with 1 cup carrot sticks and ½ cup sliced peaches in own juice.

Exchanges: 2 meats, 2 breads, 2 vegetables, 1 fruit, 1 fat

~~~~~~

Chef's Salad

1 cup dark, mixed salad greens

1 oz. cooked turkey, diced

1 tbsp. reduced-fat dressing

1 cup vegetables (broccoli, carrots, zucchini, onion, cauliflower, bell pepper), chopped

1 oz. reduced-fat Swiss cheese, diced

⅓ cup mandarin oranges

8 saltines

Exchanges: 2 meats, 2 breads, 1 vegetable, 1 fruit, 1 fat

Soup and Salad

1   serving of canned gazpacho
2   1-oz. breadsticks, topped with 2 oz. reduced-fat
    Colby jack cheese, shredded
2   plums

Exchanges: 2 meats, 2 breads, 1 vegetable, 1 fat, 1 fruit

Veggie Pizza

1   6-inch flat pita bread
¼   cup carrots, shredded
¼   cup broccoli florets
¼   cup tomatoes, diced

¼   cup prepared chunky-style
    spaghetti sauce
8   turkey pepperoni slices
1   oz. part-skim mozzarella,
    shredded

Preheat oven to 450° F. Place the bread on a cookie sheet. Spread the sauce on top of the bread. Layer with remaining ingredients, finishing with the cheese. Bake 8-10 minutes or until cheese is melted and bubbly.

Serve with 1 small orange.

Exchanges: 2 meats, 2 breads, 1 ½ vegetables, 1 fruit, 1 fat

Chicken Patty Melt

2 slices whole-grain bread, toasted and topped with 1 ounce canned white chicken meat, drained and mixed with 2 teaspoons reduced-fat mayonnaise and 1 ounce shredded part-skim mozzarella cheese. Broil open-faced until bubbly.

Serve with 1 cup celery sticks, 1 tablespoon fat-free ranch dressing and 1 medium apple.

Exchanges: 2 meats, 2 breads, 1 vegetable, 1 fruit, 1 fat

BBQ Franks and Beans

1 reduced-fat, all-beef frank, diced, mixed with 1 cup baked beans, drained, and 1 tablespoon prepared BBQ sauce. Microwave for 2-3 minutes.

Serve with 1 cup peeled and sliced cucumber tossed with 1 tablespoon lite Italian dressing and 1 cup cantaloupe cubes.

Exchanges: 2 meats, 2 breads, 1 vegetable, 1 fruit, 1 fat

Stuffed Potato

1 6-oz. potato, baked
1 oz. turkey bacon, cooked and crumbled
¼ cup tomato, diced
1 tbsp. green onions, diced
1 tsp. reduced-fat margarine
1 oz. reduced-fat cheddar cheese, shredded
¼ cup cooked broccoli florets
¼ cup mushrooms, sliced
1 tbsp. fat-free sour cream

Cut off the top of baked potato and scoop out the inside into a small bowl. Combine with remaining ingredients and mix well. Fill the shell with the mixture. Microwave until hot.

Serve with 15 grapes.
Exchanges: 2 meats, 2 breads, 1 vegetable, 1 fruit, 1 fat

Sandwich and Salad

2 slices multigrain bread
1 tsp. reduced-fat mayonnaise
2 oz. cooked turkey breast, sliced
Mustard and pickle (optional)

Serve with tossed green salad mixed with sliced tomatoes, cucumbers, carrots and peppers, 2 tablespoons fat-free salad dressing and ⅓ cup pineapple tidbits.
Exchanges: 2 meats, 2 breads, 1 vegetable, 1 fruit, 1 fat

McDonald's Happy Meal

Tossed green salad with fat-free salad dressing
Diet soda
Exchanges: 2 meats, 3 breads, 1 vegetable, 2 fats

11-oz. Frozen Dinner Entrée

1 cup fresh baby carrots
1 small apple
Exchanges: 2 meats, 2 breads, 1 vegetable, 1 fruit, 1 fat

French-Dip Roast Beef Sandwich

    1 4 oz. loaf French bread
    4 oz. lean, boneless roast beef, cooked and thinly sliced
    1 cup hot, low-sodium beef broth

Cut the bread loaf in half horizontally, then cut the pieces in half vertically to make 4 pieces. Place 2 bread pieces, cut side up, on each of 2 plates. Top each bread piece with 1 ounce roast beef and $\frac{1}{4}$ cup broth. Cover each plate with plastic wrap; microwave for 30 to 45 seconds, until heated through. Serves 2.

    Serve with 1 cup broccoli florets with 2 tablespoon reduced-fat ranch dressing and 1 cup strawberries per person.

Exchanges: 2 meats, 2 breads, 1 vegetable, 1 fruit, 1 fat

~~~~~~

Tuna Salad Pita

In small bowl, combine 4 ounce water-packed tuna, drained, $\frac{1}{4}$ cup onion, chopped and $\frac{1}{4}$ cup of celery, chopped, 2 teaspoon reduced-calorie mayonnaise and $\frac{1}{4}$ teaspoon lemon pepper seasoning. Cut one large (2 ounce) whole wheat pita in half crosswise and open to form two pockets. Fill each pocket with half of the tuna salad; top each portion of salad with $\frac{1}{4}$ cup alfalfa sprouts.

    Serve with 1 cup cucumber rounds, 1 cup carrot sticks and 15 grapes.

Exchanges: 2 meats, 2 breads, 1 vegetable, 1 fruit, 1 fat

~~~~~~

Waldorf Salad with Cheese

    1 small apple, cored and diced $\frac{1}{2}$ cup celery, chopped
    1 oz. reduced-fat cheddar cheese,   2 tsp. reduced-calorie mayonnaise
       grated

In medium bowl, combine apple, celery, cheese and mayonnaise.

    Serve over 2 cups shredded red cabbage with 3 graham crackers ($2\frac{1}{2}$-inch squares).

Exchanges: 2 meats, 2 breads, 1 vegetable, 1 fruit, 1 fat

~~~~~~

Open-Face Reuben Sandwich

2 slices reduced-calorie rye bread   ½ cup sauerkraut, drained
½ tbsp. reduced-fat Thousand Island   Black pepper, freshly ground
    dressing
1½ oz. lean corned beef, thinly sliced
½ oz. reduced-fat Swiss cheese, sliced

Preheat broiler. Lightly toast bread; spread each toast slice with 1½ teaspoon dressing. To assemble sandwiches, place toast slices, spread-side up, onto rack in broiler pan; top each with ¾ ounce corned beef, ¼ cup sauerkraut, another ¾ ounce corned beef and half of the cheese. Sprinkle evenly with pepper to taste; broil 4 inches from heat for 2 minutes until cheese is melted and lightly browned.

Veggies and mustard yogurt dip: In small bowl, combine ¼ cup plain, nonfat yogurt and 2 tablespoon prepared mustard.

Serve with ½ cup carrot sticks, ½ cup cauliflower florets and ½ cup sugar-free cherry-flavored gelatin mixed with fruit cocktail per person.
Exchanges: 2 meats, 2 breads, 1 vegetable, 1 fruit, 1 fat

~ ~

❧ DINNERS

Grilled Chicken Breasts with Corn Salsa

Salsa

1½ cups frozen corn kernels, thawed
¼ cup red onion, chopped
¼ cup red bell pepper, chopped
¼ cup fresh cilantro, chopped
1½ tbsp. fresh lime juice
4 skinless, boneless chicken
   breast halves (approx. 1 lb. each)

Chicken

½ cup cooking sherry
1 tbsp. low-sodium soy sauce
1 tbsp. fresh cilantro, chopped
2 tsp. fresh lime juice
1-2 tsp. jalapeños, chopped
   and seeded

For Salsa: Combine all ingredients in bowl. Season with salt and pepper. May be made the day before; cover and refrigerate.
For Chicken: Combine first five ingredients in medium bowl. Add chicken and turn to coat. Cover and refrigerate at least 1 hour or up to 4 hours.

    Preheat barbecue (medium-high heat) or preheat broiler. Drain chicken.

Season with salt and pepper to taste. Grill or broil chicken until just cooked through, about 4 minutes per side. Cut chicken into thin diagonal slices. Arrange chicken on plates. Top with salsa and serve.

Serve with spinach salad with sliced mushrooms and tomatoes, 1 cup cooked green beans mixed with a little salsa and a dinner roll with 1 teaspoon reduced-calorie margarine per person.

Exchanges: 3 meats, 2 breads, 2 vegetables, ½ fat

~~~~~~

Marmalade Chicken

¼ cup orange marmalade	1 tbsp. soy sauce, diluted with
¼ cup fresh lemon juice	1 tbsp. water
¼ cup white cooking wine	¼ tsp. dried thyme, crumbled
1 3-lb. chicken, cut into 8 pieces	

Combine first 5 ingredients in large bowl. Remove any visible fat, but leave skin on. Add chicken to bowl with marinade; toss to coat. Cover and refrigerate 4 hours or overnight, stirring occasionally.

Preheat oven to 400° F. Place a wire rack on top of a baking sheet. Remove chicken from marinade, reserving marinade. Place chicken skin-side up on rack. Bake 20 minutes. Turn and bake 20 minutes longer. Turn chicken skin side up and continue cooking until skin is golden brown and chicken is almost cooked through, approximately 10 minutes.

Meanwhile, boil marinade in small, heavy saucepan until reduced to glaze, about 10 minutes. Remove skin and brush chicken with glaze. Bake chicken until glaze is just set and chicken is cooked through, approximately 5 minutes. Serves 4.

Serve with 1 cup roasted potatoes, 1 cup sautéed snap peas and 1 dinner roll per person.

Exchanges: 3 meats, 2 breads, 2 vegetables, ½ fat

~~~~~~

Oriental Chicken and Cabbage Salad

1 cup canned, unsalted chicken broth	4 large garlic cloves, minced
1½ pounds skinless, boneless chicken breasts, cubed	⅓ cup rice-wine vinegar
	4 oz. snow peas, trimmed
2 tsp. jalapeño chili, seeded and minced	1 tsp. oriental sesame oil
	¼ cup fresh cilantro, chopped

1 1-gram packet sugar substitute

3 tbsp. minced fresh (or 1 tsp. ground) ginger

4½ cups red cabbage, sliced

2 cups mushrooms, sliced

1 cup green onions, chopped

2 tbsp. soy sauce, diluted with 2 tbsp. water

5½ cups Napa or green cabbage, sliced

1½ cups carrots, grated

Bring broth to simmer in heavy, large skillet over medium heat. Add chicken and simmer until just cooked through, about 7 minutes. Transfer chicken to a bowl to cool. Add snow peas to broth and cook until tender, about 3 minutes. Using slotted spoon, transfer peas to bowl of cold water. Drain. Set aside. Boil broth until reduced to ⅓ cup, about 7 minutes. Transfer to bowl; cool.

Combine vinegar, chili, cilantro, soy sauce, ginger, garlic, sesame oil and sugar substitute in medium bowl. Add broth and whisk. Place cabbage, mushrooms, carrots and onions in large bowl. Top with dressing and toss to combine. (**Note:** May be made 6 hours ahead. Cover and refrigerate.) For a colorful presentation, serve salad in red cabbage leaves. Serves 6.

Serve with ¼ cup Chinese noodles per person.

Exchanges: 3 meats, 2 breads, 2 vegetables, ½ fat

~ ~

Smoked Turkey Quesadillas

Nonstick cooking spray

6 oz. low-fat Monterey Jack cheese, grated

12 oz. 98% fat-free smoked turkey, sliced

½ tsp. ground cumin

6 7-inch low-fat flour tortillas

36 green grapes, halved lengthwise

Fresh cilantro sprigs, stemmed

1 tbsp. fresh lime juice

Coarse salt

Place tortillas on work surface. Arrange cheese, turkey, grapes and cilantro over half of each tortilla. Sprinkle with cumin. Fold tortilla over filling.

Preheat oven to 200° F. Heat large, nonstick skillet over medium heat. Coat with vegetable spray. Cook quesadillas, one at a time, until golden brown, about 3 minutes, turning once. Turn again. Brush cooked top with lime juice and sprinkle with coarse salt. Cook until golden brown, about 3 minutes. Keep warm in oven. Repeat with remaining quesadillas. Serves 6.

Serve each with ½ cup chunky salsa mixed with 1 teaspoon reduced-fat sour cream.

Exchanges: 3 meats, 2 breads, 1 vegetable, ½ fruit, 1 fat

~~~~~~

Seafood and Turkey Sausage Gumbo

¼ cup all-purpose flour

1 cup chopped onion

3 garlic cloves, chopped

1 bay leaf

1 cup canned low-salt chicken or vegetable broth

1 can (28 oz.) tomatoes in juice, diced

¼ pound small shrimp, deveined

1 tbsp. vegetable oil

1 cup green bell pepper, chopped

1 tsp. dried thyme

3 10 oz. low-fat Italian turkey casings removed

2 tsp. Creole or Cajun seasoning

2 4 oz. catfish fillets, each cut into 4 pieces

Sprinkle flour over bottom of heavy, large pot. Stir flour constantly over medium-low heat until flour turns golden brown (do not allow to burn), about 12-15 minutes. Pour browned flour into bowl.

Heat oil in same pot over medium heat. Add onion and bell pepper and sauté until tender, about 7 minutes. Add garlic, thyme and bay leaf; stir 1 minute. Add sausages and sauté until brown, breaking up with back of spoon, about 5 minutes, then add browned flour. Add tomatoes with juice, broth and Creole seasoning. Bring to boil. Reduce heat, cover and simmer 20 minutes to blend flavors, stirring frequently.

Add shrimp and catfish to pot and simmer just until seafood is opaque in center, about 5 minutes. Discard bay leaf. Season with salt and pepper and serve. Serves 4.

Serve over ½ cup steamed rice and with a green salad mixed with 2 tablespoons reduced fat dressing and 4 saltine crackers for each person.

Exchanges: 3 meats, 2 breads, 2 vegetables, 2 fats

~~~~~~

Quick Baked Fish

1½ lbs. cod, tilapia, catfish or haddock fillets

¼ cup low-fat mayonnaise

1 tsp. Dijon mustard

2 tsp. dried onion flakes

1 tsp. white wine Worcestershire sauce

1 tsp. Old Bay seasoning

¼ tsp. paprika

1 tbsp. dried (or 2 tbsp. fresh, chopped) parsley

½ tsp. lemon pepper

⅛ tsp. cayenne pepper

Nonstick cooking spray

Preheat oven to 400° F. Spray a shallow casserole with cooking spray; set aside. Wash fillets with cold water and pat dry with paper towels. Place fish fillets in prepared casserole. In a small bowl, combine remaining ingredients until well mixed. Spread mixture evenly over fillets. Bake, uncovered, for 15 minutes or until fish flakes easily with a fork. Serves 4.

Serve with steamed broccoli and ½ cup cooked brown rice and a breadstick per person.

Exchanges: 3 meats, 2 breads, 1 vegetable, 1 fat

~~~~~~

Rosemary-Sage Steak

1 lb. boneless top sirloin steak, all visible fat removed

Marinade

½ cup onion, chopped

3 tbsp. dry white cooking wine

1 tsp. olive oil

¼ tsp. salt

¼ cup fresh lemon juice

1 tbsp. Dijon mustard

½ tsp. pepper

2 tbsp. fresh (or 2 tsp. dried, crushed) rosemary, finely chopped

2 tbsp. fresh (or 2 tsp. dried) sage, finely chopped

3 medium cloves, minced, or (1 ½ tsp. bottled, minced) garlic

Put steak in an airtight plastic bag. In a small bowl, combine marinade ingredients. Pour into bag over steak and turn to coat evenly. Seal and refrigerate from 1-24 hours, turning occasionally. Preheat grill on medium-high heat. Drain steak; grill for 8-12 minutes per side, or until done to taste.

Serve with 1 cup of grilled vegetables, a 6-ounce potato topped with 1 teaspoon reduced-calorie margarine and 1 teaspoon reduced-fat sour cream per person.

Exchanges: 3 meats, 2 breads, 2 vegetables, 1 fat

~~~~~~

Grilled Sesame Chicken

2 tbsp. sesame seeds

¼ tsp. black pepper, freshly ground

2 tbsp. soy sauce, diluted with
   1½ tbsp. water

3 cloves garlic, crushed

1 tbsp. brown sugar

4 uncooked skinless chicken
   breasts

Combine all ingredients except chicken in a shallow dish. Mix well. Add chicken, turning to coat. Cover and marinate in the refrigerator for at least 2 hours. Remove chicken from the marinade. Grill 4-5 inches from medium-hot coals for 15 minutes. Turn and grill.

Serve with 1 cup cooked noodles tossed with 1 teaspoon teriyaki sauce and 1 cup sautéed oriental vegetables per person.

Exchanges: 3 meats, 2 breads, 2 vegetables, 1 fat

~~~~~~

Spicy White Bean and Chicken Chili

2 cans (16-oz.) navy beans

2 tsp. olive oil

1 extra-large onion, chopped

8 large garlic cloves, minced

½ tsp. dried oregano, crumbled

5¼ cup canned unsalted
   chicken broth

¾ lb. boneless, skinless chicken breast,
   well trimmed, cut in large pieces

¾ cup plain nonfat yogurt
   fresh cilantro, chopped

3 jalapeños, minced (optional)

1 tbsp. ground cumin

2 cans (4-oz.) green chilies, diced

4 cup water

Heat oil in large, heavy pot over medium heat. Add onion and garlic and sauté until tender, about 10 minutes. Stir in cumin and oregano and cook 1 minute. Mix in beans and chilies, then chicken broth and water. Simmer until beans are very tender and chili is creamy, about 1 hour and 45 minutes or less. (**Note:** May be made 3 days ahead. Cover and refrigerate. Reheat when ready to serve.) Ladle chili into bowls. Garnish with yogurt, cilantro and minced chilies, and serve immediately. Serves 4.

Serve with a spinach salad with reduced-calorie dressing.

Exchanges: 3 meats, 2 breads, 1 vegetable, ½ milk, 1 fat

~~~~~~

Lite Chicken Enchiladas

1 8-oz. container lite sour cream

1 10¾-oz. can Healthy Choice cream of chicken soup

1 4-oz. can green chilies, diced

12 6-inch low-fat flour tortillas

1½ cups cooked chicken, chopped

1 8 oz. container plain nonfat yogurt

1 cup 4 oz. reduced-fat cheddar cheese, shredded

¼ cup green onions, sliced

Nonstick cooking spray

Heat oven to 350° F. Spray a 13x9-inch (3-quart) baking dish with cooking spray. In medium bowl, combine sour cream, yogurt, soup and chilies; mix well. Spoon about 3 tablespoons sour-cream mixture down center of each tortilla. Reserve ¼ cup cheddar cheese; sprinkle each tortilla with remaining cheese, chicken and onions. Roll tortillas and place in spray-coated dish, seam side down. Spoon remaining sour-cream mixture over tortillas. Cover with foil and bake for 25 to 30 minutes, or until hot and bubbly. Remove foil; sprinkle with reserved ¼ cup cheese. Return to oven and bake, uncovered, an additional 5 minutes or until cheese is melted. Serves 6.

Serve enchiladas on top of shredded lettuce and chopped tomatoes with ½ cup salsa per person.

Exchanges: 3 meats, 2 breads, 1 vegetable, ½ milk, 1 fat

~ ~

Shrimp Scampi

1 lb. large fresh uncooked shrimp, deveined

1 tsp. olive oil

1 clove garlic, minced

1 tsp. margarine, melted

¼ tsp. black pepper, freshly ground

1 tbsp. fresh parsley, chopped

¼ cup white cooking wine

Combine margarine, oil, garlic, cooking wine and pepper in a large bowl. Add shrimp and toss lightly to coat. Spread shrimp in a single layer, in a shallow, oven-safe casserole dish. Broil shrimp approximately 4 inches from the heat for 3-4 minutes. Turn shrimp and broil for an additional 3-4 minutes (or until lightly browned). Sprinkle with fresh chopped parsley and serve.

Serve with Lean Cuisine Pasta Alfredo and snap peas.

Exchanges: 3 meats, 2 breads, 1 vegetable, 1 fat

~ ~

Roasted Vegetable Sandwiches

3 tbsp. balsamic or red wine vinegar

¼ cup fresh (or 1 tbsp. dried) basil, chopped

1 yellow summer squash, thinly sliced

1 red bell pepper, seeded, thinly sliced

1 small red onion, sliced and separated

8 slices sourdough bread or 4 pocket pita bread or 4 2-oz. rolls

2 tsp. olive oil

1 zucchini, thinly sliced

1 small eggplant, sliced into thin rounds

4 oz. low-fat swiss cheese, sliced

4 oz. low-fat swiss cheese, sliced

Preheat oven to 450° F. Blend vinegar, oil and basil. Add vegetables, tossing to coat. Place vegetables in roasting pan and cook, stirring occasionally, until tender and lightly browned, about 30 minutes. Cool vegetables. To assemble sandwiches, spread basil-yogurt mixture on your favorite bread, pita halves or crusty rolls. Top with cheese and fill with veggie mixture and serve.

Basil-Yogurt Spread

¼ cup plain nonfat yogurt

1 tbsp. additional fresh basil

2 tbsp. reduced-fat mayonnaise

1 tsp. lemon juice

Whisk together ingredients for spread (can be prepared ahead and refrigerated).

Exchanges: 1 meat, 2 breads, 1 ½ vegetables, 1 fat

~ ~

Argentine Corn Chicken

1 lb. boneless chicken breasts, skinless, cut into chunks

2 cloves garlic, minced

¼ tsp. leaf marjoram pepper, freshly ground, to taste

1 tbsp. canola oil

10 whole cherry tomatoes

1 large tomato, seeded, chopped

1 bay leaf

1 cup frozen whole-kernel corn, thawed

Season chicken lightly with salt and pepper. In a large, nonstick skillet, heat the oil. Add the chicken and cook until tender, turning occasionally to prevent burning. Remove from skillet and set aside; keep warm. Sauté onion and garlic in the skillet. Add chopped tomato, bay leaf and marjoram, and simmer for 10 minutes. Add corn, whole cherry tomatoes and chicken to skillet and heat through, mixing well. Serves 4.

Serve each with $\frac{1}{3}$ cup brown rice and 1 cup steamed vegetables.
Exchanges: 3 meats, 2 breads, 2 vegetables, 1 fat

~~~~~~

Green Pepper Steak

1 lb. lean sirloin steak, cut into
    $\frac{1}{4}$-inch strips
2 tbsp. all-purpose flour
$\frac{1}{4}$ tsp. pepper, freshly ground
1 can beef broth
1 medium onion, sliced

$\frac{1}{2}$ tsp. salt
1 tbsp. canola oil
1 cup canned tomatoes with juice
1 clove garlic, finely chopped
$1\frac{1}{2}$ tsp. Worcestershire sauce
1 large green pepper, cut in strips

Coat strips of round steak with flour mixed with salt and pepper. Heat oil in a large fry pan. Brown meat on all sides, drain off any fat. Add broth, tomato juice (reserving the tomato pieces for later), onion and garlic to the meat. Cover and simmer about 30-40 minutes or until meat is tender.

Add tomato pieces, green pepper strips and Worcestershire sauce. Stir and cook 10 minutes longer. Serves 4.

Serve over $\frac{1}{2}$ cup cooked rice and with 1 cup cooked carrots per person.
Exchanges: 3 meats, 2 breads, 1 vegetable, 1 fat

LEADER
DISCUSSION GUIDE

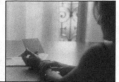

Giving Christ
First Place

Week One: Giving Christ First Place

1. Ask a volunteer to recite Matthew 6:33 from memory. Form groups of three to share what members discovered about their lives by looking at their checkbooks and calendars for the last month.

2. On the board write the headings "Lessons from the Birds" and "Lessons from the Flowers." Bring the whole group together and have someone read Matthew 6:26-28; then invite members to share what they wrote about these lessons on Day One. Have a volunteer write key ideas on the board as others share.

3. Read Luke 9:23. Have members return to their groups of three and refer to their material on Day Four, page 15. Ask them to share with their small groups what they wrote about the three commitments in Luke 9:23. Allow 10 to 12 minutes for this discussion.

4. With the whole group back together, have someone read 1 Corinthians 10:31. Explain: Our goal is to do all we do for the glory of God. Discuss how the work they are doing in the First Place program can bring glory to God.

5. In the weeks ahead, as members make progress in reaching their goals, opportunities will come to help them make a spiritual connection. Have someone read Matthew 5:16. Have two volunteers role-play a situation in which one compliments the other on weight loss. In the first case, the person makes no attempt to make a spiritual connection. In the second, the person tries to help the other see the spiritual connection.

6. Discuss the concept of using Scripture for prayer. Use examples from Day Six or Day Seven. Ask for volunteers to say a sentence prayer from their favorite Bible verse. Write this week's memory verse on the board in the form of a prayer, as on Day Seven.

7. Lead the whole group in a closing time of prayer. Ask them to thank God for the progress He will help them make in reaching their goals. Close the prayer time by asking God to use group members to bring Him glory as they deal with their health-related challenges.

Week Two: Lord, Teach Us to Pray

1. Have someone read Mark 1:35. Explain: From this snapshot of Jesus' life, we learn about His commitment to pray, His time to pray and His place to pray. Invite members to review the material on Day Two.

2. Jesus spent an exhausting day in ministry, yet He still got up early to spend time in prayer. Discuss with members why they think Jesus made that prayer time a priority. Ask volunteers to share an experience when they were tired but still decided to begin the day in prayer, describing how that decision impacted the rest of the day.

3. **Before the session**, enlist a person who you know is committed to prayer to give a testimony about the importance of prayer. Have him or her tell what time of day works best for him or her. Remind the group that in Mark 1:35, we learn that Jesus got up early to pray, but on other occasions He prayed in the evening, sometimes all night. The key is to pray when you need to pray, at a time that works for you.

4. Write the acrostic A-C-T-S vertically down the left side of the board. Ask members to recall the dimensions of prayer we associate with each letter in the acrostic. Write the words as members say them. Invite volunteers to share what they learned about their prayer lives when they considered these dimensions of prayer.

5. Explain: Often we fail to notice the conditions connected with God's promises in the Bible. Invite volunteers to share insights they gained as they studied the passages on the chart on Day One.

6. Discuss the strongholds that might keep members from reaching their goals. Ask how using God's Word can help them resist the temptations that come into their lives. Invite volunteers to recite the memory verse for this week. Discuss what this verse means in regard to their prayer lives.

7. Close in prayer by asking members to read one of the prayers they wrote in the exercise on Day Three. Tell the group you will guide the prayer time by saying, "Now let's express our adoration for God"; then give group members the opportunity to read the prayers they wrote about adoration. Continue the process with each dimension of prayer.

Week Three: The Joy of Obeying God

1. **Before the session,** write on the board the four key lessons about prayer and obedience noted on Day One. As you read each of the four principles during the meeting, pause and ask members to explain how Jesus' life demonstrated that principle.

2. Invite volunteers to share how their study of Jesus' life and His obedience impacted the way they now think about their own obedience.

3. **Before the session,** enlist someone to share a testimony about how his or her desire to obey Christ changed after becoming a Christian. Have him or her share the testimony at this point in the session. Affirm that our desire to obey God is one indication that we are Christians. Tell the group that if any members are not Christians, or are not sure they are Christians, they may talk with you following the session. Explain that they can be sure they have eternal life.

4. Form groups of three and refer members to Day Three. Ask them to share with their small group any negative thoughts they have about obeying God. Ask them to explain, if possible, the basis for these negative thoughts. In each small group, have each member read aloud two of the Positive Obedience Principles listed on page 41. Then discuss how they feel hearing those statements coming from their mouths. Ask them to consider: If they cannot do so right now, can they envision a time in the future when they could sincerely make those Positive Obedience Principles as an affirmation of personal conviction?

5. Bring the whole group back together and refer to Day Five. Ask members to think about the past week. As they worked on their First Place goals, at what point were they tempted to say "No, Lord," rather than "Yes, Lord"? Have volunteers describe their experiences.

6. Discuss how obeying God becomes an important issue in the First Place program. Insure that the group focuses on obeying God—not other people.

7. Lead the group in conversational prayers in which they use a Scripture verse as part of the prayer.

Week Four: Excuses, Excuses

1. Discuss why God gives us choices in life. If necessary, help group members focus on the fact that without real choices, we could not be

moral people capable of expressing genuine love for God. If God programmed us for certain choices, we could be functional but not moral.

2. Have a volunteer read from Psalm 1:1-3. Ask: How does God's Word influence the way we live our lives? How does God's Word affect our tendency to make excuses for our choices? Lead the group as they discuss these questions. Remind the group that God's Word tells us how to live and leaves us without excuse. We can never say, "I'm not responsible because I didn't know."

3. Form groups of four. Refer to Day Four, page 54. Invite members to share with their small groups any excuses they have used in the past concerning their lack of fitness or their indulgence in poor or unhealthy lifestyles. Discuss whether or not anyone believed their excuses. Invite members to share why they made excuses about their problems.

4. Explain: It's possible to fool other people and even fool ourselves. However, we cannot fool God. In groups of four, refer to Day Four, page 00. In the Genesis account, God asked Adam and Eve, "Do you know where you are now?" Invite members to share with their small groups where they are now in dealing with their weight problems. Are they making excuses or are they ready to assume responsibility?

5. Bring the whole group together. Write on the board: "An excuse is a lie disguised as a reason. Our enemy, Satan, stands ready to help us disguise our lies." Invite volunteers to share their past struggles to meet their goals in which they wanted to make the right choice but listened to the lie and made the wrong choice instead. Ask them to share the lies or excuses that prompted them to make the wrong choices.

6. **Before the session,** write each of the six statements from Day Five on a separate index card. Give the cards to six different people. Challenge members to assume responsibility for their lives and to begin to make right choices through God's power. Ask the card holders to read the statement on their index cards.

7. Ask members to share with others how the Scripture CDs and/or memory cards have helped them memorize Scripture. Ask members to share tips on memorizing Scripture.

8. Lead the group in a closing prayer, asking God for power to make correct choices.

Week Five: Good News About Temptation

1. **Before the session,** prepare a poster containing the statements on Day Three about our failures in resisting temptation (p. 65). Display the poster in a prominent place during the group meeting.

2. Invite three volunteers to recite 1 Corinthians 10:13 from memory.

3. Ask if group members have ever felt their struggle with health problems or unhealthy lifestyles was unique. Ask them to share if that feeling has changed since becoming part of the First Place group, and if so, why.

4. First Corinthians 10:13 describes temptation as strong and aggressive, almost like a mugger who attacks an unsuspecting victim. Invite volunteers to share an experience when the temptation to overindulge in unhealthy eating hit them with the intensity described in this passage. How did they feel? What did they do?

5. Explain: The starting point in resisting temptation is God's faithfulness, not *our* faithfulness. Refer to Day Two on page 63. Invite volunteers to share how they answered the question about God's faithfulness in helping them resist temptation.

6. Form groups of three, and have the groups discuss the following questions: How does it make you feel knowing God will not allow you to be tempted beyond what you can bear? How have you learned to prepare for temptation before the temptation occurs?

7. In the same small groups, invite them to share an experience when they were surprised by a temptation but sensed God providing an exit for them. Ask them to share with the group how they recognized the exit and how they broke free from the temptation and took God's exit.

8. Bring the whole group together. Have someone read Matthew 4:1-11. Jesus faced the pressure of temptation with Scripture. Discuss ideas for how they can use Scripture in prayer to help them resist temptation.

9. Lead the group in a closing time of prayer. Ask for volunteers to pray for their small group members that they will face and resist temptation in the coming week.

Week Six: True Satisfaction

1. On the board write the word "satisfaction." While one member writes responses, ask volunteers to suggest words or phrases that define or describe satisfaction.

2. Ask a volunteer to read Matthew 5:6. Explain: Jesus promises that those who hunger and thirst for right standing with God will be filled, or satisfied. **Before the session,** enlist someone to give a two-or-three-minute testimony focusing on how a Christian satisfies the deepest longings in his or her life by abiding in Christ. Have this person share his or her testimony at this point in the session. After the testimony, ask members to look at the box they checked on Day One (p. 76). Ask any members who are not Christians or are not sure about their relationship with Jesus to talk with you following the session.

3. **Before the session,** prepare a poster with the acrostic H-E-A-R-T written vertically down the left side. Ask members to recall the words we associate with each letter in the acrostic. Write the words on the poster as members share them (see Day Three, p. 79).

4. Invite volunteers to share how their experiences of completing the First Place Bible studies have impacted their lives. Explain that the key to enjoying the Bible as spiritual food is to add it to their lives in all the ways mentioned in the H-E-A-R-T acrostic.

5. **Before the session,** enlist a member of the group who is involved in personal ministry and finds the experience satisfying. Ask him or her to share a two-or-three-minute testimony about how doing God's work has been satisfying. Have the volunteer you enlisted before the session share at this point.

6. Explain: The song "I Can't Get No Satisfaction" describes the frustration many people feel. Ultimately, we cannot be satisfied until we deal with the spiritual need in our lives for a relationship with God. Form groups of three and ask members to share about their relationship to God or give their personal testimony. Encourage, but don't force those who may not want to share.

7. After everyone in the small groups has shared, ask them if they have used any of the Scripture memorization methods mentioned in the Bible study. Invite volunteers to share their best ideas for memorizing Scripture.

8. Close by having the small groups pray together. Encourage members to pray that God will give them satisfaction in their relationship with Him.

Week Seven: The Secret to Pleasing God

1. On the board write the words "good," "pleasing" and "perfect." Have a volunteer read Romans 12:2. Discuss how they would respond if someone offered them something described as good, pleasing and perfect. Ask them why they think some people worry about God's will for their lives.

2. Form groups of three. Refer to Day One (pp. 88-90). Invite them to discuss their answers to the questions about God's will.

3. Continue in the small groups. Explain: Romans 12:2 tells us to stop conforming to the patterns of the world. Instruct them to discuss the patterns of thinking and behaving in the world that hinder their ability to know and do God's will.

4. Bring the whole group back together. Discuss what they learned about doing God's will by studying Jesus' life on Day Three.

5. **Before the session,** make a poster with the phrase "Attitude Check" at the top. Write the six statements from Day Four (p. 96). Display this poster at this point in the session. Explain that these statements reflect the type of attitude we should develop concerning God's will. Discuss how their ability to obey God would be impacted if they developed these attitudes. Discuss how we can develop these attitudes. Remind them that the apostle Paul developed these attitudes over the course of his life; they didn't develop instantly. As we mature in Christ, we can expect these attitudes to grow and develop as well.

6. Have a volunteer read 1 Thessalonians 5:18. Explain: One way we can begin to do God's will is to develop a life characterized by thanksgiving. Discuss the difference between being thankful *in* all things and being thankful *for* all things. Remind members that we can be thankful no matter what the situation. God can work everything together for good as stated in Romans 8:28.

7. Ask several members to lead the closing time of prayer, thanking God that His will is good, pleasing and perfect. Ask God to help each group member to do His will in the week ahead.

Week Eight: Value Your Body

1. **Before the session,** prepare a poster with the seven statements included in the introduction on page 102. Label the poster: "Your Body Is
   Valuable Because . . ." Display the poster in a prominent place in the
   meeting room.

2. Ask three volunteers to quote 1 Corinthians 6:19,20 from memory.

3. Explain: The Bible uses the analogy of our bodies as temples in which
   God lives. Discuss the insights they gained in their study as a result of
   this analogy. Ask them which aspect of the beauty—physical or spiritual—of the temple was more significant and why. What application
   does this concept have for our lives as God's temples?

4. Form groups of three. Refer to Day Two (p. 105). Discuss members'
   answers about God's presence in their lives.

5. Bring the whole group back together. Have someone read Matthew
   25:14-30. Instruct members to think of principles that can be drawn
   from this passage that apply to the fact that our bodies belong to
   God. On the board write the title "On Loan from God." Appoint
   someone to record the group's responses. If the group needs help getting started, suggest the following: My body belongs to God; God
   holds me accountable for how I treat my body; God expects me to use
   my body wisely.

6. **Before the session** write the Scripture references from the chart in
   Day Four (p. 108) on slips of paper. Distribute slips to different members. Ask them to read their verses. Remind the group that our bodies
   are valuable because God has paid a high price for us.

7. Discuss how God can be honored or dishonored with our bodies.
   Refer to Day Five (pp. 109-110).

8. Close in conversational prayer using the memory verse as part of the
   prayer. Ask volunteers to thank God for the value He places on us and
   our bodies. Ask Him to help us use our bodies to honor Him.

Week Nine: Going God's Way

1. On the board write this sentence: "God, I want what You want in my
   life." Distribute index cards. Instruct members to choose a number
   between 1 and 5 that represents the degree to which they can whole-
   heartedly make this statement and mean it—1 means you struggle to

say this and mean it and 5 means you can say this without reservation. After everyone has written his or her number, invite volunteers to hold up their cards and share with the group why they chose the number they wrote.

2. Ask members to review the box they checked on Day One (p. 115). Invite volunteers to share their choices and explain why that choice is significant in their lives.

3. Have a volunteer read Psalm 51:12. Discuss what members think David was asking God to give him when he asked for a "willing spirit." Discuss how their work in the First Place program would change if God gave them willing spirits.

4. Form groups of three and have groups review the material for Day Four. Have them discuss the seriousness of having a rebellious spirit. Tell them to prepare to report to the whole group ways the teaching on rebelliousness applies to the work we are doing in the First Place program.

5. With the whole group back together, have each small group report. Then affirm that an attitude of stubbornness and rebellion can undermine the progress people can make in the First Place program.

6. Give members time to share with the whole group their struggles in going God's way. Allow time for group members to affirm and encourage them.

7. Share a personal testimony about how you learned that going God's way is the best way.

8. Invite members to share how they are progressing with memorizing Scripture. Ask volunteers to share memorized Scripture.

9. Close with a time of conversational prayer. Invite volunteers to pray that the group members will have willing spirits that long to follow God's direction.

Week Ten: Without Love—Nothing

1. Explain: Everything we know about true love is based on the love God has modeled for us. Refer to Day One (p. 129) and have someone read Ephesians 3:17-19. Ask volunteers to share what they wrote about the different aspects of God's love.

2. Invite members to share which box they checked in the exercise from Day Five (p. 137) and explain the reason for their selections. Form pairs and ask them to share with their partner what they wrote in the exercises from Day Four (pp. 134-135).

3. Bring the whole group together. Ask volunteers to recite this week's memory verse. Have someone read 1 John 4:11. Discuss the connection between God's love for us and the love we should show other people.

4. Explain: First Corinthians 13:1-3 reminds us that nothing we do in life matters if it is not done with love. Guide the group to evaluate the special challenges that come with the First Place program. Focus on the challenge of working on their health goals while continuing to deal lovingly with the people in their lives. Give members a chance to share their frustrations about this issue. Encourage others to offer practical suggestions that have helped them face and overcome this problem.

5. Ask members to think back over the 10 weeks that they have shared together. Discuss: What truth learned during this period stands out as being truly significant for them? What point marked a real breakthrough in helping them move towards specific goals?

6. Encourage members to express thanks to those in the group who have been especially helpful to them. Ask them to share with the group what others have done and why it was significant.

7. Have someone read 1 Corinthians 13. Remind the group that from God's perspective it's more important that we become loving people than that we reach health and lifestyle goals.

8. Invite volunteers to share how they have used Scripture in their prayers for this 13-week session. Ask them to share what memorizing and praying Scripture has meant to them. Close with a time of prayer. Thank God for the work He has done in their lives over the last 10 weeks.

COMMITMENT RECORDS

How to Fill Out a Commitment Record

The Commitment Record (CR) is an aid for you in keeping track of your accomplishments. Begin a new CR on the morning of the day your class meets. This ensures that your CR is complete before your next meeting. Turn in the CR weekly to your leader.

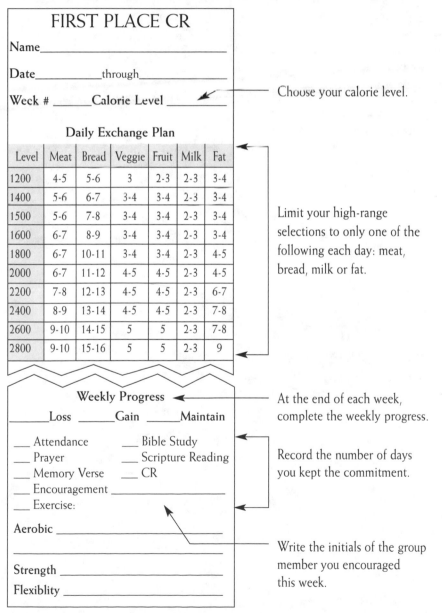

FIRST PLACE CR

Name_____

Date_____through_____

Week # _____Calorie Level _____

Choose your calorie level.

Daily Exchange Plan

Level	Meat	Bread	Veggie	Fruit	Milk	Fat
1200	4-5	5-6	3	2-3	2-3	3-4
1400	5-6	6-7	3-4	3-4	2-3	3-4
1500	5-6	7-8	3-4	3-4	2-3	3-4
1600	6-7	8-9	3-4	3-4	2-3	3-4
1800	6-7	10-11	3-4	3-4	2-3	4-5
2000	6-7	11-12	4-5	4-5	2-3	4-5
2200	7-8	12-13	4-5	4-5	2-3	6-7
2400	8-9	13-14	4-5	4-5	2-3	7-8
2600	9-10	14-15	5	5	2-3	7-8
2800	9-10	15-16	5	5	2-3	9

Limit your high-range selections to only one of the following each day: meat, bread, milk or fat.

Weekly Progress

_____Loss _____Gain _____Maintain

At the end of each week, complete the weekly progress.

___ Attendance   ___ Bible Study
___ Prayer   ___ Scripture Reading
___ Memory Verse   ___ CR
___ Encouragement_____
___ Exercise:

Record the number of days you kept the commitment.

Aerobic _____

_____

Strength _____

Flexiblity _____

Write the initials of the group member you encouraged this week.

DAY 7: Date_____

Morning _____
_____
_____

Midday _____
_____
_____

Evening _____
_____
_____

Snacks _____
_____
_____

___ Meat _____   ☐ Prayer
___ Bread _____   ☐ Bible Study
___ Vegetable _____   ☐ Scripture Reading
___ Fruit _____   ☐ Memory Verse
___ Milk _____   ☐ Encouragement
___ Fat _____   ☐ Water_____

Exercise:

Aerobic _____
_____

Strength _____

Flexibility _____

List the foods you have eaten. On this condensed CR it is not necessary to exchange each food choice. It will be the responsibility of each member that the tally marks you list below are accurate regarding each food choice. If you are unsure of an exchange, check the Live-It section of your copy of the *Member's Guide*.

List the daily food exchange choices to the left of the food groups.

Use tally marks for the actual food and water consumed.

Check off commitments completed. Use tally marks to record each 8-oz. serving of water.

List type and duration of exercise.

FIRST PLACE CR

Name_____

Date_____ through _____

Week # _____ Calorie Level _____

Daily Exchange Plan

Level	Meat	Bread	Veggie	Fruit	Milk	Fat
1200	4-5	5-6	3	2-3	2-3	3-4
1400	5-6	6-7	3-4	3-4	2-3	3-4
1500	5-6	7-8	3-4	3-4	2-3	3-4
1600	6-7	8-9	3-4	3-4	2-3	3-4
1800	6-7	10-11	3-4	3-4	2-3	4-5
2000	6-7	11-12	4-5	4-5	2-3	4-5
2200	7-8	12-13	4-5	4-5	2-3	6-7
2400	8-9	13-14	4-5	4-5	2-3	7-8
2600	9-10	14-15	5	5	2-3	7-8
2800	9-10	15-16	5	5	2-3	9

You may always choose the high range of vegetables and fruits. Limit your high range selections to only one of the following: meat, bread, milk or fat.

_____ Loss _____ Gain _____ Maintain

_____ Attendance _____ Bible Study
_____ Prayer _____ Scripture Reading
_____ Memory Verse _____ CR
_____ Encouragement
_____ Exercise
Aerobic _____

Strength _____
Flexibility _____

DAY 7: Date_____

Morning _____

Midday _____

Evening _____

Snacks _____

Meat _____ ☐ Prayer
Bread _____ ☐ Bible Study
Vegetable _____ ☐ Scripture Reading
Fruit _____ ☐ Memory Verse
Milk _____ ☐ Encouragement
Fat _____ ☐ Water
Exercise
Aerobic _____

Strength _____
Flexibility _____

DAY 6: Date_____

Morning _____

Midday _____

Evening _____

Snacks _____

Meat _____ ☐ Prayer
Bread _____ ☐ Bible Study
Vegetable _____ ☐ Scripture Reading
Fruit _____ ☐ Memory Verse
Milk _____ ☐ Encouragement
Fat _____ ☐ Water
Exercise
Aerobic _____

Strength _____
Flexibility _____

DAY 5: Date_____

Morning _____

Midday _____

Evening _____

Snacks _____

Meat _____ ☐ Prayer
Bread _____ ☐ Bible Study
Vegetable _____ ☐ Scripture Reading
Fruit _____ ☐ Memory Verse
Milk _____ ☐ Encouragement
Fat _____ ☐ Water
Exercise
Aerobic _____

Strength _____
Flexibility _____

DAY 1: Date _____

Morning _____

Midday _____

Evening _____

Snacks _____

___ Meat ___	☐ Prayer
___ Bread ___	☐ Bible Study
___ Vegetable ___	☐ Scripture Reading
___ Fruit ___	☐ Memory Verse
___ Milk ___	☐ Encouragement
___ Fat ___	___ Water ___

Exercise
Aerobic _____

Strength _____
Flexibility _____

DAY 2: Date _____

Morning _____

Midday _____

Evening _____

Snacks _____

___ Meat ___	☐ Prayer
___ Bread ___	☐ Bible Study
___ Vegetable ___	☐ Scripture Reading
___ Fruit ___	☐ Memory Verse
___ Milk ___	☐ Encouragement
___ Fat ___	___ Water ___

Exercise
Aerobic _____

Strength _____
Flexibility _____

DAY 3: Date _____

Morning _____

Midday _____

Evening _____

Snacks _____

___ Meat ___	☐ Prayer
___ Bread ___	☐ Bible Study
___ Vegetable ___	☐ Scripture Reading
___ Fruit ___	☐ Memory Verse
___ Milk ___	☐ Encouragement
___ Fat ___	___ Water ___

Exercise
Aerobic _____

Strength _____
Flexibility _____

DAY 4: Date _____

Morning _____

Midday _____

Evening _____

Snacks _____

___ Meat ___	☐ Prayer
___ Bread ___	☐ Bible Study
___ Vegetable ___	☐ Scripture Reading
___ Fruit ___	☐ Memory Verse
___ Milk ___	☐ Encouragement
___ Fat ___	___ Water ___

Exercise
Aerobic _____

Strength _____
Flexibility _____

Name

Date _____ through _____

Week # _____ Calorie Level _____

Daily Exchange Plan

Level	Meat	Bread	Veggie	Fruit	Milk	Fat
1200	4-5	5-6	3	2-3	2-3	3-4
1400	5-6	6-7	3-4	3-4	2-3	3-4
1500	5-6	7-8	3-4	3-4	2-3	3-4
1600	6-7	8-9	3-4	3-4	2-3	3-4
1800	6-7	10-11	3-4	3-4	2-3	4-5
2000	6-7	11-12	4-5	4-5	2-3	4-5
2200	7-8	12-13	4-5	4-5	2-3	6-7
2400	8-9	13-14	4-5	4-5	2-3	7-8
2600	9-10	14-15	5	5	2-3	7-8
2800	9-10	15-16	5	5	2-3	9

You may always choose the high range of vegetables and fruits. Limit your high range selections to only one of the following: meat, bread, milk or fat.

_____ Loss _____ Gain _____ Maintain

_____ Attendance _____ Bible Study
_____ Prayer _____ Scripture Reading
_____ Memory Verse _____ CR
_____ Encouragement
_____ Exercise
_____ Aerobic

_____ Strength
_____ Flexibility

DAY 7: Date _____

Morning

Midday

Evening

Snacks

_____ Meat   ☐ Prayer
_____ Bread   ☐ Bible Study
_____ Vegetable   ☐ Scripture Reading
_____ Fruit   ☐ Memory Verse
_____ Milk   ☐ Encouragement
_____ Fat   ☐ Water

Exercise
Aerobic

Strength
Flexibility

DAY 6: Date _____

Morning

Midday

Evening

Snacks

_____ Meat   ☐ Prayer
_____ Bread   ☐ Bible Study
_____ Vegetable   ☐ Scripture Reading
_____ Fruit   ☐ Memory Verse
_____ Milk   ☐ Encouragement
_____ Fat   ☐ Water

Exercise
Aerobic

Strength
Flexibility

DAY 5: Date _____

Morning

Midday

Evening

Snacks

_____ Meat   ☐ Prayer
_____ Bread   ☐ Bible Study
_____ Vegetable   ☐ Scripture Reading
_____ Fruit   ☐ Memory Verse
_____ Milk   ☐ Encouragement
_____ Fat   ☐ Water

Exercise
Aerobic

Strength
Flexibility

DAY 1: Date _____

Morning _____

Midday _____

Evening _____

Snacks _____

- ☐ Prayer
- ☐ Bible Study
- ☐ Scripture Reading
- ☐ Memory Verse
- ☐ Encouragement

____ Meat   ____ Bread   ____ Vegetable   ____ Fruit   ____ Milk   ____ Fat   ____ Water

Exercise
Aerobic _____
Strength _____
Flexibility _____

DAY 2: Date _____

Morning _____

Midday _____

Evening _____

Snacks _____

- ☐ Prayer
- ☐ Bible Study
- ☐ Scripture Reading
- ☐ Memory Verse
- ☐ Encouragement

____ Meat   ____ Bread   ____ Vegetable   ____ Fruit   ____ Milk   ____ Fat   ____ Water

Exercise
Aerobic _____
Strength _____
Flexibility _____

DAY 3: Date _____

Morning _____

Midday _____

Evening _____

Snacks _____

- ☐ Prayer
- ☐ Bible Study
- ☐ Scripture Reading
- ☐ Memory Verse
- ☐ Encouragement

____ Meat   ____ Bread   ____ Vegetable   ____ Fruit   ____ Milk   ____ Fat   ____ Water

Exercise
Aerobic _____
Strength _____
Flexibility _____

DAY 4: Date _____

Morning _____

Midday _____

Evening _____

Snacks _____

- ☐ Prayer
- ☐ Bible Study
- ☐ Scripture Reading
- ☐ Memory Verse
- ☐ Encouragement

____ Meat   ____ Bread   ____ Vegetable   ____ Fruit   ____ Milk   ____ Fat   ____ Water

Exercise
Aerobic _____
Strength _____
Flexibility _____

FIRST PLACE CR

Name _____

Date _____ through _____

Week # _____ Calorie Level _____

Daily Exchange Plan

Level	Meat	Bread	Veggie	Fruit	Milk	Fat
1200	4-5	5-6	3	2-3	2-3	3-4
1400	5-6	6-7	3-4	3-4	2-3	3-4
1500	5-6	7-8	3-4	3-4	2-3	3-4
1600	6-7	8-9	3-4	3-4	2-3	3-4
1800	6-7	10-11	3-4	3-4	2-3	4-5
2000	6-7	11-12	4-5	4-5	2-3	4-5
2200	7-8	12-13	4-5	4-5	2-3	6-7
2400	8-9	13-14	4-5	4-5	2-3	7-8
2600	9-10	14-15	5	5	2-3	7-8
2800	9-10	15-16	5	5	2-3	9

You may always choose the high range of vegetables and fruits. Limit your high range selections to only one of the following: meat, bread, milk or fat.

_____ Loss _____ Gain _____ Maintain

_____ Attendance   _____ Bible Study
_____ Prayer   _____ Scripture Reading
_____ Memory Verse   _____ CR
_____ Encouragement
_____ Exercise
Aerobic _____
Strength _____
Flexibility _____

DAY 5: Date _____

Morning _____

Midday _____

Evening _____

Snacks _____

_____ Meat   ☐ Prayer
_____ Bread   ☐ Bible Study
_____ Vegetable   ☐ Scripture Reading
_____ Fruit   ☐ Memory Verse
_____ Milk   ☐ Encouragement
_____ Fat   ☐ Water

Exercise
Aerobic _____

Strength _____
Flexibility _____

DAY 6: Date _____

Morning _____

Midday _____

Evening _____

Snacks _____

_____ Meat   ☐ Prayer
_____ Bread   ☐ Bible Study
_____ Vegetable   ☐ Scripture Reading
_____ Fruit   ☐ Memory Verse
_____ Milk   ☐ Encouragement
_____ Fat   ☐ Water

Exercise
Aerobic _____

Strength _____
Flexibility _____

DAY 7: Date _____

Morning _____

Midday _____

Evening _____

Snacks _____

_____ Meat   ☐ Prayer
_____ Bread   ☐ Bible Study
_____ Vegetable   ☐ Scripture Reading
_____ Fruit   ☐ Memory Verse
_____ Milk   ☐ Encouragement
_____ Fat   ☐ Water

Exercise
Aerobic _____

Strength _____
Flexibility _____

DAY 1: Date _____

Morning _____

Midday _____

Evening _____

Snacks _____

_____ Meat   ☐ Prayer
_____ Bread   ☐ Bible Study
_____ Vegetable   ☐ Scripture Reading
_____ Fruit   ☐ Memory Verse
_____ Milk   ☐ Encouragement
_____ Fat _____ Water

Exercise
Aerobic _____
Strength _____
Flexibility _____

DAY 2: Date _____

Morning _____

Midday _____

Evening _____

Snacks _____

_____ Meat   ☐ Prayer
_____ Bread   ☐ Bible Study
_____ Vegetable   ☐ Scripture Reading
_____ Fruit   ☐ Memory Verse
_____ Milk   ☐ Encouragement
_____ Fat _____ Water

Exercise
Aerobic _____
Strength _____
Flexibility _____

DAY 3: Date _____

Morning _____

Midday _____

Evening _____

Snacks _____

_____ Meat   ☐ Prayer
_____ Bread   ☐ Bible Study
_____ Vegetable   ☐ Scripture Reading
_____ Fruit   ☐ Memory Verse
_____ Milk   ☐ Encouragement
_____ Fat _____ Water

Exercise
Aerobic _____
Strength _____
Flexibility _____

DAY 4: Date _____

Morning _____

Midday _____

Evening _____

Snacks _____

_____ Meat   ☐ Prayer
_____ Bread   ☐ Bible Study
_____ Vegetable   ☐ Scripture Reading
_____ Fruit   ☐ Memory Verse
_____ Milk   ☐ Encouragement
_____ Fat _____ Water

Exercise
Aerobic _____
Strength _____
Flexibility _____

FIRST PLACE CR

Name _____

Date _____ through _____

Week # _____ Calorie Level _____

Daily Exchange Plan

Level	Meat	Bread	Veggie	Fruit	Milk	Fat
1200	4-5	5-6	3	2-3	2-3	3-4
1400	5-6	6-7	3-4	3-4	2-3	3-4
1500	5-6	7-8	3-4	3-4	2-3	3-4
1600	6-7	8-9	3-4	3-4	2-3	3-4
1800	6-7	10-11	3-4	3-4	2-3	4-5
2000	5-7	11-12	4-5	4-5	2-3	4-5
2200	7-8	12-13	4-5	4-5	2-3	6-7
2400	8-9	13-14	4-5	4-5	2-3	7-8
2600	9-10	14-15	5	5	2-3	7-8
2800	9-10	15-16	5	5	2-3	9

You may always choose the high range of vegetables and fruits. Limit your high range selections to only one of the following: meat, bread, milk or fat.

_____ Loss _____ Gain _____ Maintain

_____ Attendance _____ Bible Study
_____ Prayer _____ Scripture Reading
_____ Memory Verse _____ CR
_____ Encouragement
_____ Exercise
_____ Aerobic

_____ Strength
_____ Flexibility

DAY 5: Date _____

Morning _____

Midday _____

Evening _____

Snacks _____

_____ Meat   ☐ Prayer
_____ Bread   ☐ Bible Study
_____ Vegetable   ☐ Scripture Reading
_____ Fruit   ☐ Memory Verse
_____ Milk   ☐ Encouragement
_____ Fat   _____ Water

Exercise
Aerobic _____

Strength _____
Flexibility _____

DAY 6: Date _____

Morning _____

Midday _____

Evening _____

Snacks _____

_____ Meat   ☐ Prayer
_____ Bread   ☐ Bible Study
_____ Vegetable   ☐ Scripture Reading
_____ Fruit   ☐ Memory Verse
_____ Milk   ☐ Encouragement
_____ Fat   _____ Water

Exercise
Aerobic _____

Strength _____
Flexibility _____

DAY 7: Date _____

Morning _____

Midday _____

Evening _____

Snacks _____

_____ Meat   ☐ Prayer
_____ Bread   ☐ Bible Study
_____ Vegetable   ☐ Scripture Reading
_____ Fruit   ☐ Memory Verse
_____ Milk   ☐ Encouragement
_____ Fat   _____ Water

Exercise
Aerobic _____

Strength _____
Flexibility _____

DAY 1: Date _____

Morning _____

Midday _____

Evening _____

Snacks _____

Meat _____	☐ Prayer
Bread _____	☐ Bible Study
Vegetable _____	☐ Scripture Reading
Fruit _____	☐ Memory Verse
Milk _____	☐ Encouragement
Fat _____	Water _____

Exercise
Aerobic _____

Strength _____

Flexibility _____

DAY 2: Date _____

Morning _____

Midday _____

Evening _____

Snacks _____

Meat _____	☐ Prayer
Bread _____	☐ Bible Study
Vegetable _____	☐ Scripture Reading
Fruit _____	☐ Memory Verse
Milk _____	☐ Encouragement
Fat _____	Water _____

Exercise
Aerobic _____

Strength _____

Flexibility _____

DAY 3: Date _____

Morning _____

Midday _____

Evening _____

Snacks _____

Meat _____	☐ Prayer
Bread _____	☐ Bible Study
Vegetable _____	☐ Scripture Reading
Fruit _____	☐ Memory Verse
Milk _____	☐ Encouragement
Fat _____	Water _____

Exercise
Aerobic _____

Strength _____

Flexibility _____

DAY 4: Date _____

Morning _____

Midday _____

Evening _____

Snacks _____

Meat _____	☐ Prayer
Bread _____	☐ Bible Study
Vegetable _____	☐ Scripture Reading
Fruit _____	☐ Memory Verse
Milk _____	☐ Encouragement
Fat _____	Water _____

Exercise
Aerobic _____

Strength _____

Flexibility _____

Name _____

Date _____ through _____

Week # _____ Calorie Level _____

Daily Exchange Plan

Level	Meat	Bread	Veggie	Fruit	Milk	Fat
1200	4-5	5-6	3	2-3	2-3	3-4
1400	5-6	6-7	3-4	3-4	2-3	3-4
1500	5-6	7-8	3-4	3-4	2-3	3-4
1600	6-7	8-9	3-4	3-4	2-3	3-4
1800	6-7	10-11	3-4	3-4	2-3	4-5
2000	6-7	11-12	4-5	4-5	2-3	4-5
2200	7-8	12-13	4-5	4-5	2-3	6-7
2400	8-9	13-14	4-5	4-5	2-3	7-8
2600	9-10	14-15	5	5	2-3	7-8
2800	9-10	15-16	5	5	2-3	9

You may always choose the high range of vegetables and fruits. Limit your high range selections to only one of the following: meat, bread, milk or fat.

_____ Loss _____ Gain _____ Maintain

_____ Attendance _____ Bible Study
_____ Prayer _____ Scripture Reading
_____ Memory Verse _____ CR
_____ Encouragement
_____ Exercise
_____ Aerobic

_____ Strength
_____ Flexibility

DAY 5: Date _____

Morning _____

Midday _____

Evening _____

Snacks _____

_____ Meat ☐ Prayer
_____ Bread ☐ Bible Study
_____ Vegetable ☐ Scripture Reading
_____ Fruit ☐ Memory Verse
_____ Milk ☐ Encouragement
_____ Fat Water _____

Exercise
Aerobic _____

Strength _____
Flexibility _____

DAY 6: Date _____

Morning _____

Midday _____

Evening _____

Snacks _____

_____ Meat ☐ Prayer
_____ Bread ☐ Bible Study
_____ Vegetable ☐ Scripture Reading
_____ Fruit ☐ Memory Verse
_____ Milk ☐ Encouragement
_____ Fat Water _____

Exercise
Aerobic _____

Strength _____
Flexibility _____

DAY 7: Date _____

Morning _____

Midday _____

Evening _____

Snacks _____

_____ Meat ☐ Prayer
_____ Bread ☐ Bible Study
_____ Vegetable ☐ Scripture Reading
_____ Fruit ☐ Memory Verse
_____ Milk ☐ Encouragement
_____ Fat Water _____

Exercise
Aerobic _____

Strength _____
Flexibility _____

DAY 1: Date _____ **DAY 2:** Date _____ **DAY 3:** Date _____ **DAY 4:** Date _____

Each day contains the same fields:

Morning _____

Midday _____

Evening _____

Snacks _____

	Meat _____	☐ Prayer
	Bread _____	☐ Bible Study
	Vegetable _____	☐ Scripture Reading
	Fruit _____	☐ Memory Verse
	Milk _____	☐ Encouragement
	Fat _____ Water _____	

Exercise
Aerobic _____

Strength _____
Flexibility _____

FIRST PLACE CR

Name _____

Date _____ through _____

Week # _____ Calorie Level _____

Daily Exchange Plan

Level	Meat	Bread	Veggie	Fruit	Milk	Fat
1200	4-5	5-6	3	2-3	2-3	3-4
1400	5-6	6-7	3-4	3-4	2-3	3-4
1500	5-6	7-8	3-4	3-4	2-3	3-4
1600	6-7	8-9	3-4	3-4	2-3	3-4
1800	6-7	10-11	3-4	3-4	2-3	4-5
2000	6-7	11-12	4-5	4-5	2-3	4-5
2200	7-8	12-13	4-5	4-5	2-3	6-7
2400	8-9	13-14	4-5	4-5	2-3	7-8
2600	9-10	14-15	5	5	2-3	7-8
2800	9-10	15-16	5	5	2-3	9

You may always choose the high range of vegetables and fruits. Limit your high range selections to only one of the following: meat, bread, milk or fat.

_____ Loss _____ Gain _____ Maintain

_____ Attendance _____ Bible Study
_____ Prayer _____ Scripture Reading
_____ Memory Verse _____ CR
_____ Encouragement
_____ Exercise
_____ Aerobic

Strength _____
Flexibility _____

DAY 5: Date _____

Morning _____

Midday _____

Evening _____

Snacks _____

_____ Meat   ☐ Prayer
_____ Bread   ☐ Bible Study
_____ Vegetable ☐ Scripture Reading
_____ Fruit   ☐ Memory Verse
_____ Milk   ☐ Encouragement
_____ Fat   Water _____

Exercise
Aerobic _____

Strength _____
Flexibility _____

DAY 6: Date _____

Morning _____

Midday _____

Evening _____

Snacks _____

_____ Meat   ☐ Prayer
_____ Bread   ☐ Bible Study
_____ Vegetable ☐ Scripture Reading
_____ Fruit   ☐ Memory Verse
_____ Milk   ☐ Encouragement
_____ Fat   Water _____

Exercise
Aerobic _____

Strength _____
Flexibility _____

DAY 7: Date _____

Morning _____

Midday _____

Evening _____

Snacks _____

_____ Meat   ☐ Prayer
_____ Bread   ☐ Bible Study
_____ Vegetable ☐ Scripture Reading
_____ Fruit   ☐ Memory Verse
_____ Milk   ☐ Encouragement
_____ Fat   Water _____

Exercise
Aerobic _____

Strength _____
Flexibility _____

DAY 1: Date _____

Morning _____
_____
_____

Midday _____
_____
_____

Evening _____
_____
_____

Snacks _____
_____
_____

____ Meat   ☐ Prayer
____ Bread   ☐ Bible Study
____ Vegetable   ☐ Scripture Reading
____ Fruit   ☐ Memory Verse
____ Milk   ☐ Encouragement
____ Fat   ____ Water

Exercise
Aerobic _____
Strength _____
Flexibility _____

DAY 2: Date _____

Morning _____
_____
_____

Midday _____
_____
_____

Evening _____
_____
_____

Snacks _____
_____
_____

____ Meat   ☐ Prayer
____ Bread   ☐ Bible Study
____ Vegetable   ☐ Scripture Reading
____ Fruit   ☐ Memory Verse
____ Milk   ☐ Encouragement
____ Fat   ____ Water

Exercise
Aerobic _____
Strength _____
Flexibility _____

DAY 3: Date _____

Morning _____
_____
_____

Midday _____
_____
_____

Evening _____
_____
_____

Snacks _____
_____
_____

____ Meat   ☐ Prayer
____ Bread   ☐ Bible Study
____ Vegetable   ☐ Scripture Reading
____ Fruit   ☐ Memory Verse
____ Milk   ☐ Encouragement
____ Fat   ____ Water

Exercise
Aerobic _____
Strength _____
Flexibility _____

DAY 4: Date _____

Morning _____
_____
_____

Midday _____
_____
_____

Evening _____
_____
_____

Snacks _____
_____
_____

____ Meat   ☐ Prayer
____ Bread   ☐ Bible Study
____ Vegetable   ☐ Scripture Reading
____ Fruit   ☐ Memory Verse
____ Milk   ☐ Encouragement
____ Fat   ____ Water

Exercise
Aerobic _____
Strength _____
Flexibility _____

Name _____

Date _____ through _____

Week # _____ Calorie Level _____

Daily Exchange Plan

Level	Meat	Bread	Veggie	Fruit	Milk	Fat
1200	4-5	5-6	3	2-3	2-3	3-4
1400	5-6	6-7	3-4	3-4	2-3	3-4
1500	5-6	7-8	3-4	3-4	2-3	3-4
1600	6-7	8-9	3-4	3-4	2-3	3-4
1800	6-7	10-11	3-4	3-4	2-3	4-5
2000	6-7	11-12	4-5	4-5	2-3	4-5
2200	7-8	12-13	4-5	4-5	2-3	6-7
2400	8-9	13-14	4-5	4-5	2-3	7-8
2600	9-10	14-15	5	5	2-3	7-8
2800	9-10	15-16	5	5	2-3	9

You may always choose the high range of vegetables and fruits. Limit your high range selections to only one of the following: meat, bread, milk or fat.

_____ Loss _____ Gain _____ Maintain

_____ Attendance _____ Bible Study
_____ Prayer _____ Scripture Reading
_____ Memory Verse _____ CR
_____ Encouragement
_____ Exercise
_____ Aerobic

Strength _____
Flexibility _____

DAY 5: Date _____

Morning _____
_____

Midday _____
_____

Evening _____
_____

Snacks _____
_____

_____ Meat   ☐ Prayer
_____ Bread   ☐ Bible Study
_____ Vegetable   ☐ Scripture Reading
_____ Fruit   ☐ Memory Verse
_____ Milk   ☐ Encouragement
_____ Fat   Water _____

Exercise _____
Aerobic _____

Strength _____
Flexibility _____

DAY 6: Date _____

Morning _____
_____

Midday _____
_____

Evening _____
_____

Snacks _____
_____

_____ Meat   ☐ Prayer
_____ Bread   ☐ Bible Study
_____ Vegetable   ☐ Scripture Reading
_____ Fruit   ☐ Memory Verse
_____ Milk   ☐ Encouragement
_____ Fat   Water _____

Exercise _____
Aerobic _____

Strength _____
Flexibility _____

DAY 7: Date _____

Morning _____
_____

Midday _____
_____

Evening _____
_____

Snacks _____
_____

_____ Meat   ☐ Prayer
_____ Bread   ☐ Bible Study
_____ Vegetable   ☐ Scripture Reading
_____ Fruit   ☐ Memory Verse
_____ Milk   ☐ Encouragement
_____ Fat   Water _____

Exercise _____
Aerobic _____

Strength _____
Flexibility _____

DAY 1: Date _____   **DAY 2:** Date _____   **DAY 3:** Date _____   **DAY 4:** Date _____

Morning _____

Midday _____

Evening _____

Snacks _____

Meat ___	☐ Prayer
Bread ___	☐ Bible Study
Vegetable ___	☐ Scripture Reading
Fruit ___	☐ Memory Verse
Milk ___	☐ Encouragement
Fat ___	Water ___

Exercise
Aerobic _____
Strength _____
Flexibility _____

Morning _____

Midday _____

Evening _____

Snacks _____

Meat ___	☐ Prayer
Bread ___	☐ Bible Study
Vegetable ___	☐ Scripture Reading
Fruit ___	☐ Memory Verse
Milk ___	☐ Encouragement
Fat ___	Water ___

Exercise
Aerobic _____
Strength _____
Flexibility _____

Morning _____

Midday _____

Evening _____

Snacks _____

Meat ___	☐ Prayer
Bread ___	☐ Bible Study
Vegetable ___	☐ Scripture Reading
Fruit ___	☐ Memory Verse
Milk ___	☐ Encouragement
Fat ___	Water ___

Exercise
Aerobic _____
Strength _____
Flexibility _____

Morning _____

Midday _____

Evening _____

Snacks _____

Meat ___	☐ Prayer
Bread ___	☐ Bible Study
Vegetable ___	☐ Scripture Reading
Fruit ___	☐ Memory Verse
Milk ___	☐ Encouragement
Fat ___	Water ___

Exercise
Aerobic _____
Strength _____
Flexibility _____

FIRST PLACE CR

Name _____

Date _____ through _____

Week # _____ Calorie Level _____

Daily Exchange Plan

Level	Meat	Bread	Veggie	Fruit	Milk	Fat
1200	4-5	5-6	3	2-3	2-3	3-4
1400	5-6	6-7	3-4	3-4	2-3	3-4
1500	5-6	7-8	3-4	3-4	2-3	3-4
1600	6-7	8-9	3-4	3-4	2-3	3-4
1800	6-7	10-11	3-4	3-4	2-3	4-5
2000	6-7	11-12	4-5	4-5	2-3	4-5
2200	7-8	12-13	4-5	4-5	2-3	6-7
2400	8-9	13-14	4-5	4-5	2-3	7-8
2600	9-10	14-15	5	5	2-3	7-8
2800	9-10	15-16	5	5	2-3	9

You may always choose the high range of vegetables and fruits. Limit your high range selections to only one of the following: meat, bread, milk or fat.

____ Loss ____ Gain ____ Maintain

____ Attendance ____ Bible Study
____ Prayer ____ Scripture Reading
____ Memory Verse ____ CR
____ Encouragement
____ Exercise
Aerobic _____

Strength _____
Flexibility _____

DAY 5: Date _____

Morning _____

Midday _____

Evening _____

Snacks _____

____ Meat   ☐ Prayer
____ Bread   ☐ Bible Study
____ Vegetable   ☐ Scripture Reading
____ Fruit   ☐ Memory Verse
____ Milk   ☐ Encouragement
____ Fat   Water _____

Exercise
Aerobic _____

Strength _____
Flexibility _____

DAY 6: Date _____

Morning _____

Midday _____

Evening _____

Snacks _____

____ Meat   ☐ Prayer
____ Bread   ☐ Bible Study
____ Vegetable   ☐ Scripture Reading
____ Fruit   ☐ Memory Verse
____ Milk   ☐ Encouragement
____ Fat   Water _____

Exercise
Aerobic _____

Strength _____
Flexibility _____

DAY 7: Date _____

Morning _____

Midday _____

Evening _____

Snacks _____

____ Meat   ☐ Prayer
____ Bread   ☐ Bible Study
____ Vegetable   ☐ Scripture Reading
____ Fruit   ☐ Memory Verse
____ Milk   ☐ Encouragement
____ Fat   Water _____

Exercise
Aerobic _____

Strength _____
Flexibility _____

DAY 1: Date _____

Morning _____

Midday _____

Evening _____

Snacks _____

____ Meat	☐ Prayer
____ Bread	☐ Bible Study
____ Vegetable	☐ Scripture Reading
____ Fruit	☐ Memory Verse
____ Milk	☐ Encouragement
____ Fat	
____ Water	

Exercise
Aerobic _____
Strength _____
Flexibility _____

DAY 2: Date _____

Morning _____

Midday _____

Evening _____

Snacks _____

____ Meat	☐ Prayer
____ Bread	☐ Bible Study
____ Vegetable	☐ Scripture Reading
____ Fruit	☐ Memory Verse
____ Milk	☐ Encouragement
____ Fat	
____ Water	

Exercise
Aerobic _____
Strength _____
Flexibility _____

DAY 3: Date _____

Morning _____

Midday _____

Evening _____

Snacks _____

____ Meat	☐ Prayer
____ Bread	☐ Bible Study
____ Vegetable	☐ Scripture Reading
____ Fruit	☐ Memory Verse
____ Milk	☐ Encouragement
____ Fat	
____ Water	

Exercise
Aerobic _____
Strength _____
Flexibility _____

DAY 4: Date _____

Morning _____

Midday _____

Evening _____

Snacks _____

____ Meat	☐ Prayer
____ Bread	☐ Bible Study
____ Vegetable	☐ Scripture Reading
____ Fruit	☐ Memory Verse
____ Milk	☐ Encouragement
____ Fat	
____ Water	

Exercise
Aerobic _____
Strength _____
Flexibility _____

FIRST PLACE CR

Name _____

Date _____ through _____

Week # _____ Calorie Level _____

Daily Exchange Plan

Level	Meat	Bread	Veggie	Fruit	Milk	Fat
1200	4-5	5-6	3	2-3	2-3	3-4
1400	5-6	6-7	3-4	3-4	2-3	3-4
1500	5-6	7-8	3-4	3-4	2-3	3-4
1600	6-7	8-9	3-4	3-4	2-3	3-4
1800	6-7	10-11	3-4	3-4	2-3	4-5
2000	6-7	11-12	4-5	4-5	2-3	4-5
2200	7-8	12-13	4-5	4-5	2-3	6-7
2400	8-9	13-14	4-5	4-5	2-3	7-8
2600	9-10	14-15	5	5	2-3	7-8
2800	9-10	15-16	5	5	2-3	9

You may always choose the high range of vegetables and fruits. Limit your high range selections to only one of the following: meat, bread, milk or fat.

____ Loss ____ Gain ____ Maintain

____ Attendance ____ Bible Study
____ Prayer ____ Scripture Reading
____ Memory Verse ____ CR
____ Encouragement
____ Exercise
Aerobic _____

Strength _____
Flexibility _____

DAY 5: Date _____

Morning _____

Midday _____

Evening _____

Snacks _____

____ Meat   ☐ Prayer
____ Bread   ☐ Bible Study
____ Vegetable   ☐ Scripture Reading
____ Fruit   ☐ Memory Verse
____ Milk   ☐ Encouragement
____ Fat   Water _____

Exercise
Aerobic _____

Strength _____
Flexibility _____

DAY 6: Date _____

Morning _____

Midday _____

Evening _____

Snacks _____

____ Meat   ☐ Prayer
____ Bread   ☐ Bible Study
____ Vegetable   ☐ Scripture Reading
____ Fruit   ☐ Memory Verse
____ Milk   ☐ Encouragement
____ Fat   Water _____

Exercise
Aerobic _____

Strength _____
Flexibility _____

DAY 7: Date _____

Morning _____

Midday _____

Evening _____

Snacks _____

____ Meat   ☐ Prayer
____ Bread   ☐ Bible Study
____ Vegetable   ☐ Scripture Reading
____ Fruit   ☐ Memory Verse
____ Milk   ☐ Encouragement
____ Fat   Water _____

Exercise
Aerobic _____

Strength _____
Flexibility _____

DAY 1: Date _____

Morning _____

Midday _____

Evening _____

Snacks _____

Meat ____	☐ Prayer
Bread ____	☐ Bible Study
Vegetable ____	☐ Scripture Reading
Fruit ____	☐ Memory Verse
Milk ____	☐ Encouragement
Fat ____	
Water ____	

Exercise
Aerobic _____
Strength _____
Flexibility _____

DAY 2: Date _____

Morning _____

Midday _____

Evening _____

Snacks _____

Meat ____	☐ Prayer
Bread ____	☐ Bible Study
Vegetable ____	☐ Scripture Reading
Fruit ____	☐ Memory Verse
Milk ____	☐ Encouragement
Fat ____	
Water ____	

Exercise
Aerobic _____
Strength _____
Flexibility _____

DAY 3: Date _____

Morning _____

Midday _____

Evening _____

Snacks _____

Meat ____	☐ Prayer
Bread ____	☐ Bible Study
Vegetable ____	☐ Scripture Reading
Fruit ____	☐ Memory Verse
Milk ____	☐ Encouragement
Fat ____	
Water ____	

Exercise
Aerobic _____
Strength _____
Flexibility _____

DAY 4: Date _____

Morning _____

Midday _____

Evening _____

Snacks _____

Meat ____	☐ Prayer
Bread ____	☐ Bible Study
Vegetable ____	☐ Scripture Reading
Fruit ____	☐ Memory Verse
Milk ____	☐ Encouragement
Fat ____	
Water ____	

Exercise
Aerobic _____
Strength _____
Flexibility _____

FIRST PLACE CR

Name _____

Date _____ through _____

Week # _____ Calorie Level _____

Daily Exchange Plan

Level	Meat	Bread	Veggie	Fruit	Milk	Fat
1200	4-5	5-6	3	2-3	2-3	3-4
1400	5-6	6-7	3-4	3-4	2-3	3-4
1500	5-6	7-8	3-4	3-4	2-3	3-4
1600	6-7	8-9	3-4	3-4	2-3	3-4
1800	6-7	10-11	3-4	3-4	2-3	4-5
2000	6-7	11-12	4-5	4-5	2-3	4-5
2200	7-8	12-13	4-5	4-5	2-3	6-7
2400	8-9	13-14	4-5	4-5	2-3	7-8
2600	9-10	14-15	5	5	2-3	7-8
2800	9-10	15-16	5	5	2-3	9

You may always choose the high range of vegetables and fruits. Limit your high range selections to only one of the following: meat, bread, milk or fat.

_____ Loss _____ Gain _____ Maintain

_____ Attendance _____ Bible Study
_____ Prayer _____ Scripture Reading
_____ Memory Verse _____ CR
_____ Encouragement
_____ Exercise
Aerobic _____

Strength _____
Flexibility _____

DAY 5: Date _____

Morning _____

Midday _____

Evening _____

Snacks _____

_____ Meat ☐ Prayer
_____ Bread ☐ Bible Study
_____ Vegetable ☐ Scripture Reading
_____ Fruit ☐ Memory Verse
_____ Milk ☐ Encouragement
_____ Fat ☐ Water

Exercise
Aerobic _____

Strength _____
Flexibility _____

DAY 6: Date _____

Morning _____

Midday _____

Evening _____

Snacks _____

_____ Meat ☐ Prayer
_____ Bread ☐ Bible Study
_____ Vegetable ☐ Scripture Reading
_____ Fruit ☐ Memory Verse
_____ Milk ☐ Encouragement
_____ Fat ☐ Water

Exercise
Aerobic _____

Strength _____
Flexibility _____

DAY 7: Date _____

Morning _____

Midday _____

Evening _____

Snacks _____

_____ Meat ☐ Prayer
_____ Bread ☐ Bible Study
_____ Vegetable ☐ Scripture Reading
_____ Fruit ☐ Memory Verse
_____ Milk ☐ Encouragement
_____ Fat ☐ Water

Exercise
Aerobic _____

Strength _____
Flexibility _____

DAY 1: Date _____

Morning _____

Midday _____

Evening _____

Snacks _____

Meat _____ ☐ Prayer
Bread _____ ☐ Bible Study
Vegetable _____ ☐ Scripture Reading
Fruit _____ ☐ Memory Verse
Milk _____ ☐ Encouragement
Fat _____ Water _____

Exercise
Aerobic _____
Strength _____
Flexibility _____

DAY 2: Date _____

Morning _____

Midday _____

Evening _____

Snacks _____

Meat _____ ☐ Prayer
Bread _____ ☐ Bible Study
Vegetable _____ ☐ Scripture Reading
Fruit _____ ☐ Memory Verse
Milk _____ ☐ Encouragement
Fat _____ Water _____

Exercise
Aerobic _____
Strength _____
Flexibility _____

DAY 3: Date _____

Morning _____

Midday _____

Evening _____

Snacks _____

Meat _____ ☐ Prayer
Bread _____ ☐ Bible Study
Vegetable _____ ☐ Scripture Reading
Fruit _____ ☐ Memory Verse
Milk _____ ☐ Encouragement
Fat _____ Water _____

Exercise
Aerobic _____
Strength _____
Flexibility _____

DAY 4: Date _____

Morning _____

Midday _____

Evening _____

Snacks _____

Meat _____ ☐ Prayer
Bread _____ ☐ Bible Study
Vegetable _____ ☐ Scripture Reading
Fruit _____ ☐ Memory Verse
Milk _____ ☐ Encouragement
Fat _____ Water _____

Exercise
Aerobic _____
Strength _____
Flexibility _____

Name _____

Date _____ through _____

Week # _____ Calorie Level _____

Daily Exchange Plan

Level	Meat	Bread	Veggie	Fruit	Milk	Fat
1200	4-5	5-6	3	2-3	2-3	3-4
1400	5-6	6-7	3-4	3-4	2-3	3-4
1500	5-6	7-8	3-4	3-4	2-3	3-4
1600	6-7	8-9	3-4	3-4	2-3	3-4
1800	6-7	10-11	3-4	3-4	2-3	4-5
2000	6-7	11-12	4-5	4-5	2-3	4-5
2200	7-8	12-13	4-5	4-5	2-3	6-7
2400	8-9	13-14	4-5	4-5	2-3	7-8
2600	9-10	14-15	5	5	2-3	7-8
2800	9-10	15-16	5	5	2-3	9

You may always choose the high range of vegetables and fruits. Limit your high range selections to only one of the following: meat, bread, milk or fat.

_____ Loss _____ Gain _____ Maintain

_____ Attendance _____ Bible Study
_____ Prayer _____ Scripture Reading
_____ Memory Verse _____ CR
_____ Encouragement
_____ Exercise
Aerobic _____

Strength _____
Flexibility _____

DAY 5: Date _____

Morning _____

Midday _____

Evening _____

Snacks _____

_____ Meat   ☐ Prayer
_____ Bread   ☐ Bible Study
_____ Vegetable   ☐ Scripture Reading
_____ Fruit   ☐ Memory Verse
_____ Milk   ☐ Encouragement
_____ Fat   Water _____

Exercise
Aerobic _____

Strength _____
Flexibility _____

DAY 6: Date _____

Morning _____

Midday _____

Evening _____

Snacks _____

_____ Meat   ☐ Prayer
_____ Bread   ☐ Bible Study
_____ Vegetable   ☐ Scripture Reading
_____ Fruit   ☐ Memory Verse
_____ Milk   ☐ Encouragement
_____ Fat   Water _____

Exercise
Aerobic _____

Strength _____
Flexibility _____

DAY 7: Date _____

Morning _____

Midday _____

Evening _____

Snacks _____

_____ Meat   ☐ Prayer
_____ Bread   ☐ Bible Study
_____ Vegetable   ☐ Scripture Reading
_____ Fruit   ☐ Memory Verse
_____ Milk   ☐ Encouragement
_____ Fat   Water _____

Exercise
Aerobic _____

Strength _____
Flexibility _____

DAY 1: Date _____

Morning _____

Midday _____

Evening _____

Snacks _____
_____

___ Meat ___	☐ Prayer
___ Bread ___	☐ Bible Study
___ Vegetable ___	☐ Scripture Reading
___ Fruit ___	☐ Memory Verse
___ Milk ___	☐ Encouragement
___ Fat ___ Water ___	

Exercise
Aerobic _____
Strength _____
Flexibility _____

DAY 2: Date _____

Morning _____

Midday _____

Evening _____

Snacks _____
_____

___ Meat ___	☐ Prayer
___ Bread ___	☐ Bible Study
___ Vegetable ___	☐ Scripture Reading
___ Fruit ___	☐ Memory Verse
___ Milk ___	☐ Encouragement
___ Fat ___ Water ___	

Exercise
Aerobic _____
Strength _____
Flexibility _____

DAY 3: Date _____

Morning _____

Midday _____

Evening _____

Snacks _____
_____

___ Meat ___	☐ Prayer
___ Bread ___	☐ Bible Study
___ Vegetable ___	☐ Scripture Reading
___ Fruit ___	☐ Memory Verse
___ Milk ___	☐ Encouragement
___ Fat ___ Water ___	

Exercise
Aerobic _____
Strength _____
Flexibility _____

DAY 4: Date _____

Morning _____

Midday _____

Evening _____

Snacks _____
_____

___ Meat ___	☐ Prayer
___ Bread ___	☐ Bible Study
___ Vegetable ___	☐ Scripture Reading
___ Fruit ___	☐ Memory Verse
___ Milk ___	☐ Encouragement
___ Fat ___ Water ___	

Exercise
Aerobic _____
Strength _____
Flexibility _____

FIRST PLACE CR

Name _____

Date _____ through _____

Week # _____ Calorie Level _____

Daily Exchange Plan

Level	Meat	Bread	Veggie	Fruit	Milk	Fat
1200	4-5	5-6	3	2-3	2-3	3-4
1400	5-6	6-7	3-4	3-4	2-3	3-4
1500	5-6	7-8	3-4	3-4	2-3	3-4
1600	6-7	8-9	3-4	3-4	2-3	3-4
1800	6-7	10-11	3-4	3-4	2-3	4-5
2000	6-7	11-12	4-5	4-5	2-3	4-5
2200	7-8	12-13	4-5	4-5	2-3	6-7
2400	8-9	13-14	4-5	4-5	2-3	7-8
2600	9-10	14-15	5	5	2-3	7-8
2800	9-10	15-16	5	5	2-3	9

You may always choose the high range of vegetables and fruits. Limit your high range selections to only one of the following: meat, bread, milk or fat.

____ Loss   ____ Gain   ____ Maintain

____ Attendance   ____ Bible Study
____ Prayer   ____ Scripture Reading
____ Memory Verse   ____ CR
____ Encouragement
____ Exercise
____ Aerobic

____ Strength
____ Flexibility

DAY 5: Date _____

Morning _____

Midday _____

Evening _____

Snacks _____

____ Meat
____ Bread
____ Vegetable
____ Fruit
____ Milk
____ Fat

☐ Prayer
☐ Bible Study
☐ Scripture Reading
☐ Memory Verse
☐ Encouragement
____ Water

Exercise _____
Aerobic _____

Strength _____
Flexibility _____

DAY 6: Date _____

Morning _____

Midday _____

Evening _____

Snacks _____

____ Meat
____ Bread
____ Vegetable
____ Fruit
____ Milk
____ Fat

☐ Prayer
☐ Bible Study
☐ Scripture Reading
☐ Memory Verse
☐ Encouragement
____ Water

Exercise _____
Aerobic _____

Strength _____
Flexibility _____

DAY 7: Date _____

Morning _____

Midday _____

Evening _____

Snacks _____

____ Meat
____ Bread
____ Vegetable
____ Fruit
____ Milk
____ Fat

☐ Prayer
☐ Bible Study
☐ Scripture Reading
☐ Memory Verse
☐ Encouragement
____ Water

Exercise _____
Aerobic _____

Strength _____
Flexibility _____

DAY 1: Date _____

Morning _____

Midday _____

Evening _____

Snacks _____

- _____ Meat
- _____ Bread
- _____ Vegetable
- _____ Fruit
- _____ Milk
- _____ Fat

- ☐ Prayer
- ☐ Bible Study
- ☐ Scripture Reading
- ☐ Memory Verse
- ☐ Encouragement
- _____ Water

Exercise

Aerobic _____

Strength _____

Flexibility _____

DAY 2: Date _____

Morning _____

Midday _____

Evening _____

Snacks _____

- _____ Meat
- _____ Bread
- _____ Vegetable
- _____ Fruit
- _____ Milk
- _____ Fat

- ☐ Prayer
- ☐ Bible Study
- ☐ Scripture Reading
- ☐ Memory Verse
- ☐ Encouragement
- _____ Water

Exercise

Aerobic _____

Strength _____

Flexibility _____

DAY 3: Date _____

Morning _____

Midday _____

Evening _____

Snacks _____

- _____ Meat
- _____ Bread
- _____ Vegetable
- _____ Fruit
- _____ Milk
- _____ Fat

- ☐ Prayer
- ☐ Bible Study
- ☐ Scripture Reading
- ☐ Memory Verse
- ☐ Encouragement
- _____ Water

Exercise

Aerobic _____

Strength _____

Flexibility _____

DAY 4: Date _____

Morning _____

Midday _____

Evening _____

Snacks _____

- _____ Meat
- _____ Bread
- _____ Vegetable
- _____ Fruit
- _____ Milk
- _____ Fat

- ☐ Prayer
- ☐ Bible Study
- ☐ Scripture Reading
- ☐ Memory Verse
- ☐ Encouragement
- _____ Water

Exercise

Aerobic _____

Strength _____

Flexibility _____

FIRST PLACE CR

Name _____

Date _____ through _____

Week # _____ Calorie Level _____

Daily Exchange Plan

Level	Meat	Bread	Veggie	Fruit	Milk	Fat
1200	4-5	5-6	3	2-3	2-3	3-4
1400	5-6	6-7	3-4	3-4	2-3	3-4
1500	5-6	7-8	3-4	3-4	2-3	3-4
1600	6-7	8-9	3-4	3-4	2-3	3-4
1800	6-7	10-11	3-4	3-4	2-3	4-5
2000	6-7	11-12	4-5	4-5	2-3	4-5
2200	7-8	12-13	4-5	4-5	2-3	6-7
2400	8-9	13-14	4-5	4-5	2-3	7-8
2600	9-10	14-15	5	5	2-3	7-8
2800	9-10	15-16	5	5	2-3	9

You may always choose the high range of vegetables and fruits. Limit your high range selections to only one of the following: meat, bread, milk or fat.

_____ Loss _____ Gain _____ Maintain

_____ Attendance _____ Bible Study
_____ Prayer _____ Scripture Reading
_____ Memory Verse _____ CR
_____ Encouragement
_____ Exercise
Aerobic _____

Strength _____
Flexibility _____

DAY 5: Date _____

Morning _____

Midday _____

Evening _____

Snacks _____

_____ Meat ☐ Prayer
_____ Bread ☐ Bible Study
_____ Vegetable ☐ Scripture Reading
_____ Fruit ☐ Memory Verse
_____ Milk ☐ Encouragement
_____ Fat _____ Water

Exercise
Aerobic _____

Strength _____
Flexibility _____

DAY 6: Date _____

Morning _____

Midday _____

Evening _____

Snacks _____

_____ Meat ☐ Prayer
_____ Bread ☐ Bible Study
_____ Vegetable ☐ Scripture Reading
_____ Fruit ☐ Memory Verse
_____ Milk ☐ Encouragement
_____ Fat _____ Water

Exercise
Aerobic _____

Strength _____
Flexibility _____

DAY 7: Date _____

Morning _____

Midday _____

Evening _____

Snacks _____

_____ Meat ☐ Prayer
_____ Bread ☐ Bible Study
_____ Vegetable ☐ Scripture Reading
_____ Fruit ☐ Memory Verse
_____ Milk ☐ Encouragement
_____ Fat _____ Water

Exercise
Aerobic _____

Strength _____
Flexibility _____

DAY 1: Date _____

Morning _____

Midday _____

Evening _____

Snacks _____

___ Meat	☐ Prayer
___ Bread	☐ Bible Study
___ Vegetable	☐ Scripture Reading
___ Fruit	☐ Memory Verse
___ Milk	☐ Encouragement
___ Fat ___ Water	

Exercise
Aerobic _____

Strength _____
Flexibility _____

DAY 2: Date _____

Morning _____

Midday _____

Evening _____

Snacks _____

___ Meat	☐ Prayer
___ Bread	☐ Bible Study
___ Vegetable	☐ Scripture Reading
___ Fruit	☐ Memory Verse
___ Milk	☐ Encouragement
___ Fat ___ Water	

Exercise
Aerobic _____

Strength _____
Flexibility _____

DAY 3: Date _____

Morning _____

Midday _____

Evening _____

Snacks _____

___ Meat	☐ Prayer
___ Bread	☐ Bible Study
___ Vegetable	☐ Scripture Reading
___ Fruit	☐ Memory Verse
___ Milk	☐ Encouragement
___ Fat ___ Water	

Exercise
Aerobic _____

Strength _____
Flexibility _____

DAY 4: Date _____

Morning _____

Midday _____

Evening _____

Snacks _____

___ Meat	☐ Prayer
___ Bread	☐ Bible Study
___ Vegetable	☐ Scripture Reading
___ Fruit	☐ Memory Verse
___ Milk	☐ Encouragement
___ Fat ___ Water	

Exercise
Aerobic _____

Strength _____
Flexibility _____

CONTRIBUTORS

Jody Wilkinson, M.D., M.S., the writer of the Wellness Worksheets for this study, is a physician and exercise physiologist at the Cooper Institute in Dallas, Texas. He trained at the University of Texas Health Science Center in San Antonio, Texas, and Baylor University Medical Center in Dallas. Dr. Wilkinson conducts research on physical activity, nutrition and weight management and has worked with the American Heart Association to develop a health program. He believes strongly in using biblical teaching to motivate people to take care of their physical bodies and enjoy abundant living. Jody and his wife, Natalie, have been married 10 years and have two daughters, Jordan and Sarah, and twin sons, Joel and Cooper.

Scott Wilson, C.E.C., A.A.C., the author of the menu plans in this study, has been cooking professionally for 23 years. A certified executive chef with the American Culinary Federation, he currently works in the Greater Atlanta area as a personal chef and food consultant. Along with serving as the national food consultant for First Place, he is a chef/spokesperson for Yves's Veggie Cuisine of Vancouver, British Columbia, a part-time nutrition teacher at Life University and chef/host of a cable cooking show in the Atlanta area, Cooking 4 Life. Scott has also authored two cookbooks, *Dining Under the Magnolia* and *Healthy Home Cooking*. In his spare time, he is active in church work and spends time with his wife, Jennifer, and their daughter, Katie.

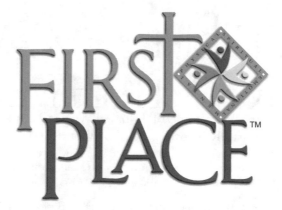

First Place was founded under the providence of God and with the conviction that there is a need for a program which will train the minds, develop the moral character and enrich the spiritual lives of all those who may come within the sphere of its influence.

First Place is dedicated to providing quality information for development of a physical, emotional and spiritual environment leading to a life that honors God in Jesus Christ. As a health-oriented program, First Place will stress the highest excellence and proficiency in instruction with a goal of developing within each participant mastery of all the basics of a lasting healthy lifestyle, so that all may achieve their highest potential in body, mind and spirit. The spiritual development of each participant shall be given high priority so that each may come to the knowledge of Jesus Christ and God's plan and purpose for each life.

First Place offers instruction, encouragement and support to help members experience a more abundant life. Please contact the First Place national office in Houston, Texas at (800) 727-5223 for information on the following resources:

❖ Training Opportunities

❖ Conferences/Rallies

❖ Workshops

❖ Fitness Weeks

Send personal testimonies to:

First Place

7401 Katy Freeway
Houston, TX 77024

Phone: **(800) 727-5223**
Website: ***www.firstplace.org***

THE BIBLE'S WAY TO WEIGHT LOSS

First Place—the Bible-Based Weight-Loss Program
Used Successfully by over a Half Million People!

Are you one of the millions of disheartened dieters who've tried one fad diet after another without success? If so, your search for a successful diet is over! First Place is the proven weight-loss program born over 20 years ago in the First Baptist Church of Houston.

But First Place does much more than help you take off weight and keep it off. This Bible-based program will transform your life in every way—physically, mentally, spiritually and emotionally. Now's the time to join!

ESSENTIAL FIRST PLACE PROGRAM MATERIALS

Group Leaders need:

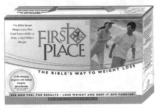

• Group Starter Kit
ISBN 08307.28708

This kit has everything group leaders need to help others change their lives forever by giving Christ first place!

Kit includes:

- *Leader's Guide*
- *Member's Guide*
- *Giving Christ First Place Bible Study* with Scripture Memory Music CD
- *Choosing to Change* by Carole Lewis
- *First Place* by Carole Lewis with Terry Whalin
- *Orientation* Video
- *Nine Commitments* Video
- *Food Exchange Plan* Video

Group Members need:

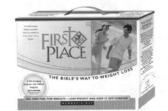

• Member's Kit
ISBN 08307.28694

All the material is easy to understand and spells out principles members can easily apply in their daily lives.

Kit includes:

- *Member's Guide*
- *Choosing to Change* by Carole Lewis
- 13 Commitment Records
- Four Motivational Audiocassettes
- *Prayer Journal*
- Scripture Memory Verses: *Walking in the Word*

• First Place Bible Study

Giving Christ First Place Bible Study with Scripture Memory Music CD

Bible Study
ISBN 08307.28643

Other Bible studies available

Available at your local Christian bookstore or by calling 1-800-4-GOSPEL.
Join the First Place community at **www.firstplace.org**

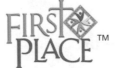

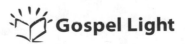

11063

Bible Studies
to Help You Put Christ
First

Scripture Memory Music CD's Inside Each Study

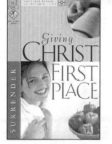

Giving Christ First Place
Bible Study
ISBN 08307.28643

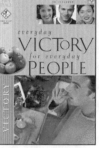

Everyday Victory for Everyday People
Bible Study
ISBN 08307.28651

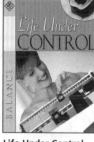

Life Under Control
Bible Study
ISBN 08307.29305

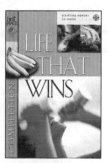

Life That Wins
Bible Study
ISBN 08307.29240

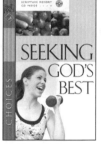

Seeking God's Best
Bible Study
ISBN 08307.29259

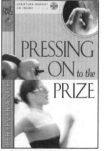

Pressing On to the Prize
Bible Study
ISBN 08307.29267

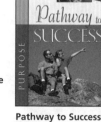

Pathway to Success
Bible Study
ISBN 08307.29275

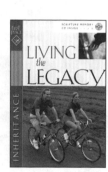

Living the Legacy
Bible Study
ISBN 08307.29283

Available at your local Christian bookstore or by calling 1-800-4-GOSPEL.

Join the First Place community at www.firstplace.org

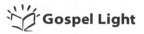 Gospel Light

11062

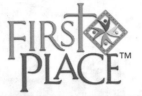

Available from your local Gospel Light supplier

First Place Resource Order Form

TITLE	ISBN/SPCN	QTY	PRICE	ITEM TOTAL
First Place Group Starter Kit ($198 Value!)	08307.28708		149.99	
First Place Member's Kit ($101 Value!)	08307.28694		79.99	
First Place (Lewis/Whalin) (included in Group Starter Kit)	08307.28635		18.99	
Choosing to Change (Lewis) (included in Member's and Group Starter Kits)	08307.28627		8.99	
Giving Christ First Place Bible Study w/Scripture Memory CD (included in Group Starter Kit)	08307.28643		19.99	
Everyday Victory for Everyday People Bible Study w/Scripture Memory CD	08307.28651		19.99	
Life That Wins Bible Study w/ Scripture Memory CD	08307.29240		19.99	
Life Under Control Bible Study w/ Scripture Memory CD	08307.29305		19.99	
Pressing On to the Prize Bible Study w/ Scripture Memory CD	08307.29267		19.99	
Seeking God's Best Bible Study w/ Scripture Memory CD	08307.29259		19.99	
Living the Legacy Bible Study w/ Scripture Memory CD	08307.29283		19.99	
Pathway to Success Bible Study w/ Scripture Memory CD	08307.29275		19.99	
Prayer Journal (included in Member's Kit)	08307.29003		9.99	
Motivational Audiocassettes (pkg. of 4) (included in Member's Kit)	607135.005988		29.99	
Commitment Records (pkg. o f 13) (included in Member's Kit)	08307.29011		6.99	
Scripture Memory Verses: Walking in the Word (included in Member's Kit)	08307.28996		14.99	
Leader's Guide (included in Group Starter Kit)	08307.28678		19.99	
Food Exchange Plan Video (included in Group Starter Kit)	607135.006138		29.99	
Orientation Video (included in Group Starter Kit)	607135.005940		29.99	
Nine Commitments Video (included in Group Starter Kit)	607135.005957		39.99	
Giving Christ First Place Scripture Memory Music CD	607135.005902		9.99	
Giving Christ First Place Scripture Memory Music Cassette	607135.005919		6.99	
Everyday Victory for Everyday People Scripture Memory Music CD	607135.005926		9.99	
Everyday Victory for Everyday People Scripture Memory Music Cassette	607135.005933		6.99	
Life Under Control Scripture Memory Music CD	607135.006213		9.99	
Life Under Control Scripture Memory Music Cassette	607135.006206		6.99	
Life That Wins Scripture Memory Music CD	607135.006237		9.99	
Life That Wins Scripture Memory Music Cassette	607135.006220		6.99	
Seeking God's Best Scripture Memory Music CD	607135.006244		9.99	
Seeking God's Best Scripture Memory Music Cassette	607135.006251		6.99	
Pressing On to the Prize Scripture Memory Music CD	607135.006268		9.99	
Pressing On to the Prize Scripture Memory Music Cassette	607135.006275		6.99	
Pathway to Success Scripture Memory Music CD	607135.006282		9.99	
Pathway to Success Scripture Memory Music Cassette	607135.006299		6.99	
Living the Legacy Scripture Memory Music CD	607135.006305		9.99	
Living the Legacy Scripture Memory Music Cassette	607135.006312		6.99	

PRICES SUBJECT TO CHANGE.

Total : $_____

Inspiration
&Information
Every Month!
Subscribe Today!

Every newsletter gives you:

- **New recipes**

- **Helpful articles**

- **Food tips**

- **Inspiring testimonies**

- **Coming events**

- **And much more!**

**A Must-Have Publication for All First Place
Leaders & Members!**

Register for our FREE
e-newsletter at
www.firstplace.org

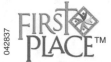

042837

www.firstplace.org

Great Reading for Your Spiritual and Physical Health!

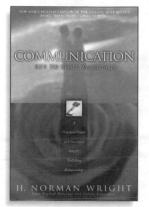

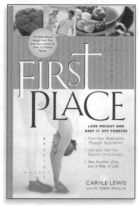

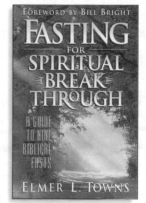

Communication: Key to Your Marriage
H. Norman Wright
A practical guide to creating a happy, fulfilling relationship

Paperback
ISBN 08307.25334

First Place
By Carole Lewis with Terry Whalin
Complete guide to losing weight the healthy way

Hardcover
ISBN 08307.28635

Fasting for Spiritual Breakthrough
Elmer L. Towns
Nine biblical fasts to strengthen your faith

Paperback
ISBN 08307.18397

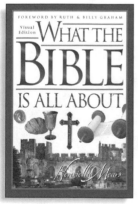

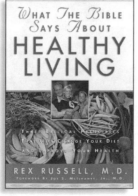

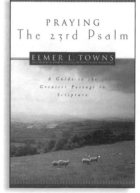

What the Bible Is All About Visual Edition
Henrietta Mears
Over 500 full-color photographs and illustrations

Hardcover
ISBN 08307.24311

What the Bible Says About Healthy Living
Rex Russell, M.D.
Three biblical principles that will change your diet and improve your health.

Paperback
ISBN 08307.18583

Praying the 23rd Psalm
Elmer L. Towns
Great devotional reading that will bring comfort and peace to believers

Paperback
ISBN 08307.27760

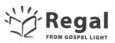

Regal
FROM GOSPEL LIGHT

Available at your local Christian bookstore. www.regalbooks.com